Evidence-Based Dentistry

An Introduction

Evidence-Based Dentistry
An Introduction

Allan K. Hackshaw
Deputy-Director
Cancer Research UK and UCL Cancer Trials Centre
University College London

Elizabeth A. Paul
Lecturer in Epidemiology and Medical Statistics
Cancer Research UK and UCL Cancer Trials Centre
University College London

Elizabeth S. Davenport
Professor of Dental Education
Barts and The London School of Medicine and Dentistry
Queen Mary, University of London

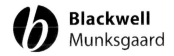

Blackwell
Munksgaard

© 2006 Allan Hackshaw
Blackwell Munksgaard, a Blackwell Publishing Company

Editorial offices:
Blackwell Publishing Ltd, 9600 Garsington Road, Oxford OX4 2DQ, UK
   Tel: +44 (0)1865 776868
Blackwell Publishing Professional, 2121 State Avenue, Ames, Iowa 50014-8300, USA
   Tel: +1 515 292 0140
Blackwell Publishing Asia, 550 Swanston Street, Carlton, Victoria 3053, Australia
   Tel: +61 (0)3 8359 1011

First published 2006 by Blackwell Munksgaard
2   2007

ISBN: 978-1-4051-2496-6

Library of Congress Cataloging-in-Publication Data

Hackshaw, Allan K.
   Evidence-based dentistry : an introduction / Allan K. Hackshaw, Elizabeth A. Paul, Elizabeth S. Davenport.
      p. ; cm.
   Includes index.
   ISBN-13: 978-1-4051-2496-6 (pbk. : alk. paper)
   ISBN-10: 1-4051-2496-2 (pbk. : alk. paper)
1. Evidence-based dentistry.   2. Dentistry–Miscellanea.   3. Evidence-based medicine.
   [DNLM: 1. Dental Research.   2. Evidence-Based Medicine. WU 20.5 H123e 2006]
I. Paul, Elizabeth A.   II. Davenport, Elizabeth S.   III. Title.

   RK53.H33 2006
   617.6–dc22

                                                                      2005035491

A catalogue record for this title is available from the British Library

Set in 10/12pt Palatino & Futura
by TechBooks
Printed and bound in Singapore
by Markono Print Media Pte Ltd

For further information on Blackwell Publishing, visit our website:
www.blackwellmunksgaard.com

Contents

Foreword

Attitudes have changed dramatically over the last twenty years. Both patients and practitioners want to know more about the treatments given and the agents that put us at risk of disease. Will a treatment work? Is this the best available treatment? Can anything be done to prevent a particular disease? Dentists may meet people who have read a news item and want to know if it applies to them. Or we open the mail to find a flyer from a drug company advertising a new dental material or nutritional supplement. Should we ignore the flyer or not?

The ability to answer these questions is inherently dependent upon the ability to read and interpret the dental literature. This is why it has become increasingly important for students and practitioners to be proficient in the area of evidence-based dentistry and critical appraisal. The purpose of this book is to allow dentists to gain confidence in their own ability to assess research reports and overcome the misconception that the conclusions of an article are correct simply because it has been published.

This book is beautifully written and presented. Above all it is simple to read and achieves great clarity through basing discussion of concepts on relevant papers from the literature. It will enable students and practitioners to gain the knowledge they need to assess and make use of the ever increasing amount of research information available to them.

The book makes a major contribution by providing dental professionals with skills that will allow them to practice evidence based dentistry. In so doing it will enable practitioners to be more confident about the basis on which they make clinical decisions and provide advice to those for whom they have responsibility. Encouraging readers to adopt the skills described in the book will lead to improvement of dental health care.

Elizabeth Treasure
Professor of Dental Public Health, Cardiff

Preface

During the years spent as a dental student and while practising as a dentist, it is important to be able to identify risk factors and causes of disease and to assess whether methods of detection, prevention and treatment are effective or not. Throughout their careers, dentists need to know where to obtain information on the management and treatment of patients and interpret this information correctly. They also need to keep abreast of new developments and techniques. Combining this knowledge with clinical experience is essentially **evidence-based dentistry**. Information can be found in research articles in journals, in textbooks and in reports from professional bodies. There is, however, an abundance of published research and it can be difficult for the student or dentist to interpret articles and decide whether these would be useful in their work. The ability to do this is central to practising evidence-based dentistry and this book aims to provide an introduction to understanding and interpreting research papers.

Several textbooks are available on evidence-based medicine and they discuss issues that are also relevant to evidence-based dentistry. They tend to concentrate on giving an overview of the topic and its underlying purpose, rather than the basic understanding of the interpretation of research results. The intention of this book is to develop the skills of interpretation of results and provide an understanding of the strengths and limitations of different approaches to research. It is aimed at dental undergraduates, postgraduates and dental practitioners.

There is always a quantitative element to research and many people find the numerical aspects of research daunting. This is often because their introduction to the measures most frequently used in research papers is through algebra. For some people, mathematical formulae can obscure rather than clarify simple concepts. It is vital that dentists understand the quantitative aspects of research papers because the fundamental findings of much of the research in dentistry depend on the interpretation of the data. Discussing examples of the *use* of particular techniques, rather than the algebra that underlies them, can lead to a better understanding of the information conveyed by statistical results.

This book introduces the basic epidemiological and statistical aspects of research as a means to assist the dentist in reading and understanding scientific reports. The book is not meant to be a reference text, but rather a guide to interpreting published research. The layout has been designed for the reader to go through each chapter in turn because they build on key ideas. All the topics and concepts covered are based entirely on published papers from dental journals, and the understanding of numerical concepts is achieved through building on particular examples.

Chapter 1 summarises the purpose of evidence-based dentistry. Chapters 2 and 3 provide an introduction to some fundamental concepts used in the subsequent chapters. These chapters make an important distinction between research based on counting people and research based on taking measurements on people. Chapter 4 uses these concepts to show how comparisons are made between groups of people. This allows us to assess the effectiveness of new treatments (covered in Chapter 5) or identify risk factors for or causes of oral disease (covered in Chapter 6). Chapter 7 shows how to examine methods of detecting oral disease. Chapters 2, 5, 6 and 7 cover the main types of research study: namely, prevalence (or cross-sectional) studies, randomised trials, cohort studies and case–control studies. Chapter 8 compares and contrasts these different study designs. Chapter 9 provides an introduction to systematic reviews, which involves combining the information from *several* studies.

Chapters 2, 5, 6, 7 and 9 are each based on a full published paper from a dental journal, sometimes supplemented with parts of other papers. Each paragraph of the paper is numbered to allow the reader to pinpoint easily the particular section being discussed. Chapter 3 is based on results found in a published article (without reproducing any part of it).

These chapters are composed in a similar way. They address the following questions, which provide a structured approach to reading research articles or commercial product information:

- What is the specific aim of the study (identifying the research question)?
- What are the outcome measures or interventions?
- How was the study conducted (assessing aspects of the study design)?
- What are the main results and how do we interpret them?
- How good is the evidence?
- What does the study contribute to dental practice?

Although the concepts covered in each chapter are discussed in the context of a single study, they apply to any similar study. Because evidence-based dentistry is based on interpreting research articles, we use them as teaching tools rather than present the concepts first followed by examples. Our intention is not to critically appraise the articles but to use them to illustrate research methods and statistical ideas in dentistry. We hope that our approach makes it easier for the reader to understand the points we are trying to get across by relating them to specific examples of research.

This book is not intended to provide a comprehensive text on how to undertake research in dentistry, but rather serve as an introduction to understanding published research. Details of how to perform statistical tests and analyses commonly found in the literature are not presented here. Most statistical analyses are now performed by computers and it is not necessary to know how to do the calculations. It is the interpretation of the results of the analysis that matters. A number of simple algebraic formulae are given because these may assist some readers in understanding basic concepts. Readers who find algebra a deterrent can ignore the formulae; they are not essential in developing the concepts. A reading list is given at the end of the book for those wishing to learn more about research methodology.

We have attempted to provide a broad range of articles that between them represent much of what is to be found in the dental literature or provided by dental company representatives. The book should provide a foundation on which to base the practice of evidence-based dentistry. The book is built on a course that Allan Hackshaw and Elizabeth Paul developed and delivered to dental students at Barts and The London School of Dentistry, where Elizabeth Davenport is Professor of Dental Education.

Acknowledgements

The authors and publishers are grateful to the copyright holders who have kindly given us permission for the journal material to be reproduced here for illustrative purposes. Our thanks are extended to:

Macmillan (*British Dental Journal*)
Elsevier (*Journal of Dentistry*)
American Medical Association (*Archives of Otolaryngology—Head & Neck Surgery*)
International and American Associations of Dental Research (*Journal of Dental Research*)
John Wiley & Sons Ltd (*The Cochrane Library*)

Evidence-based dentistry: what it is and how to practise it

Oral disease is widespread and most people, from children to the elderly, will seek dental care at some point, either for a check-up or for treatment following clinical symptoms. More people are living longer and more will retain most or all of their teeth. For example, in 1978, 30% of adults in the UK had lost all of their teeth compared with 13% in 1998; complete tooth loss usually occurs over the age of 45 years[1]. Furthermore, changing diets and lifestyles affect patterns of oral disease and there are constantly new advances in treatments. All of these have important implications for effective dental care management.

About 45% of the population aged 18 years and over are registered with a National Health Service (NHS) dental practitioner in England and Wales[2]. In a survey of UK general dental practitioners in 2000 an estimated 85% of all patients were seen in the NHS and 15% privately, though this varies greatly across the UK[3]. Other studies suggest that as many as 25% of patients are seen privately[3]. Dental care can be expensive. In 2001–2002, general dentistry in the UK generated an estimated income of £3.7 billion[4]. Patients spent a total of £2.5 billion of which about £1.9 billion was spent privately and £0.6 billion was spent on NHS charges[4]. Dentists therefore have an obligation to provide the most effective treatment available and use the best methods of disease prevention and diagnosis while taking financial cost and their expertise into consideration.

WHAT IS EVIDENCE-BASED DENTISTRY?

In dentistry there are well-established causes of oral disease, and diagnostic methods and treatments that work. There is also bad practice: there may be tests and treatments that are effective but not commonly used and, possibly worse, tests and treatments that despite being ineffective are used. How can we decide what is a cause of disease and what is not, and what is an effective treatment and what is ineffective?

Evidence-based dentistry is the integration and interpretation of the available current research evidence, combined with personal experience. It allows dentists, as well as academic researchers, to keep abreast of new developments and to make decisions that should improve their clinical practice. The term 'evidence-based medicine', from which evidence-based dentistry has followed, is relatively new (it first became current in the early 1990s) but the core principles that underlie the subject have been in place for many decades in the areas of epidemiology and public health.

The American Dental Association has defined evidence-based dentistry as[5]:

> *an approach to oral health care that requires the judicious integration of:*
>
> - *systematic assessments of clinically relevant scientific evidence, relating to the patient's oral and medical condition and history, together with the*
> - *dentist's clinical expertise and*
> - *the patient's treatment needs and preferences*

WHY DO WE NEED EVIDENCE-BASED DENTISTRY?

Graduates from dental schools are up to date with the best practice in dentistry current at the time they graduate. Some of this knowledge gradually becomes out of date as new information and technology appear. It is important, especially with regards to patient safety, for dentists to be able to keep up to date with developments in diagnosis, prevention and treatment of oral disease, and newly discovered causes of disease.

There is an overwhelming amount of evidence that comes from research and policy-making organisations, but there is no one organisation that synthesises and assesses all this evidence. Advances in dentistry are usually first reported in dental journals, and in order to keep up with new research, healthcare professionals need to feel confident that they can read and evaluate dental papers. Keeping abreast of new developments through reading current literature can seem onerous and hard to combine with a heavy clinical workload. Fortunately, having an understanding of how to interpret research results, and some practice in reading the literature in a structured way, can turn the dental literature into a useful and comprehensible practice tool.

Consider the following two examples:

- Cigarette smoking is a cause of periodontitis. Why is it that not everyone who smokes develops periodontitis? Why do some non-smokers develop periodontitis? Given these two observations, how can we say that smoking is a cause of this disorder?
- Acute ulcerative gingivitis can be treated with the antibiotic metronidazole. Why is it that not every patient given metronidazole recovers from the disease? Why do some untreated patients recover? Given this, how can we say that metronidazole is an effective treatment?

Both of the above examples illustrate that people are naturally variable in their responses to exposures or treatments. Different people respond to the same exposure, or same treatment, in different ways.

When examining causes and treatments of disease we always see variation between people in whether they are affected by an exposure or treatment. We need to be able to judge whether any differences observed are due entirely to natural variation or an effect that is above and beyond that of natural variation. For example, if 100 patients with acute ulcerative gingivitis were treated with metronidazole and 95 recovered, would this be sufficient information to say that metronidazole worked? To answer this we would also need to be able to answer the question, 'What recovery rate would we expect if they had not been treated?'. Suppose that in a similar group of untreated patients only 10 recovered. Then the effect of metronidazole above that of natural variation is associated with an *extra* 85 patients who recover. We may consider this difference to be large enough to allow us to say that metronidazole is effective. Similarly, to determine whether smoking is a cause of periodontitis or not, we could observe how many smokers develop the disease, but we also need to ask, 'How many non-smokers would develop periodontitis?'.

Clinical research allows us to make decisions about causes of and treatments for disease, while allowing for the natural differences between people. Evidence-based dentistry is founded on clinical research.

HOW TO PRACTICE EVIDENCE-BASED DENTISTRY

Evidence-based dentistry is built upon asking questions. These could arise in several ways:

- Those instigated by the management of a single patient. You may be interested in someone who has presented with clinical symptoms or wish to provide advice on some aspect of prevention (for example, you have diagnosed a patient with gingivitis, how best can this be treated?).
- A patient would like some information from you about some aspect of dentistry (for example, should they use a manual or electric toothbrush?).
- You may be interested in a particular topic which you have discussed with a colleague or you have read about in journals or other media (for example, a colleague tells you that there is a new treatment for periodontitis, and you wish to find out more about this).

The following sections describe the main steps in practising evidence-based dentistry.

(1) Define the question

Regardless of what prompted you to search for information, the next step is to define the question clearly. Is the aim sensible? Is it appropriate for the management of patients? Will it have an impact on your practice? These are all questions to consider when formulating the question because they will help you to focus not only on the literature search but also on the interpretation of the information found.

In any one day a dentist may be faced with any of the following situations:

SCENARIO 1: BEST TOOTHBRUSH

A middle-aged woman who has arthritis in her hands attends the dental practice for a routine check-up and says she has read an article about tooth brushing. She particularly wants to know whether she should be using an electric toothbrush instead of a conventional manual one. Could you advise her?

Questions

(1) What are the options for tooth brushing?
(2) Which are more effective, electric or manual toothbrushes?
(3) If electric toothbrushes are more effective, is any one better than the others? There are different types (for example rotary or sonic) and different manufacturers.

SCENARIO 2: FLUORIDE SUPPLEMENTATION

Jenny's mother comes to your surgery asking whether or not she should give her daughter fluoride supplements. Jenny is 3 years old and is at high risk of developing dental caries.

Questions

(1) What is the rationale for using fluoride in the prevention of dental caries?
(2) What are the options for delivering fluoride?
(3) What alternatives would be effective and appropriate for a 3-year-old child?
(4) What are the side effects of using fluoride supplements?

SCENARIO 3: BACTERIAL ENDOCARDITIS

An adult who has a congenital cardiac lesion is at high risk of developing bacterial endocarditis. He requires dental care including root canal treatment and the extraction of several teeth. There is some doubt in your mind about whether penicillin prophylaxis is warranted for this individual.

Questions

(1) What type of congenital cardiac lesion does he have?
(2) What is the occurrence of bacterial endocarditis in the population?

(3) What is the risk of developing bacterial endocarditis as a result of invasive dental treatment?

(4) What are the guidelines for prophylaxis against bacterial endocarditis?

(5) What is the efficacy of antibiotic prophylaxis?

(6) What are the potential benefits and harms of any such prophylaxis?

The scenarios presented above illustrate some of the types of questions which can be addressed through evidence-based dentistry. The purpose of your search will fall into one or more of the following categories of research:

- Monitoring and surveillance of oral health and disease
- Identifying causes of disease or risk factors associated with disease
- Detecting and diagnosing disease
- Preventing disease
- Evaluating treatments for disease

(2) Search for the information

There are many sources of information on dental treatments and on causes of oral disease. Published articles in medical and dental journals are now easy to search on-line, using electronic databases such as Medline. Organisations such as the National Institute for Clinical Excellence produce summaries of the evidence on particular therapies and guidelines about their use. You may also be contacted by dental company representatives who provide literature on their products. Details of the main information sources are provided in Chapter 9.

The evidence found in the literature will come from various types of study, employing different methodologies:

- Observational studies
  - Cross-sectional survey
  - Cohort study
  - Case–control study
- Interventional studies
  - Clinical trial
- Reviews
  - Systematic reviews
  - Narrative reviews

The original research papers will be either observational or interventional studies, and, in Chapters 2–7 the methodology and interpretation of each of these types of study are discussed in relation to an example from a published paper. Chapter 8 compares and contrasts observational and interventional study designs. Reviews of the literature on a particular topic can provide an overview of the research that has been published in that area. However, it is still essential to understand the findings from the individual studies that make up a review. Chapter 9 suggests approaches to finding and synthesising evidence, and introduces the topic of systematic reviews.

(3) Interpret the evidence

This is the most time-consuming step and is often seen as the most difficult aspect of reading research papers. However, understanding how to interpret results is central to evaluating the evidence yourself. When reading a research article, many people rely on the conclusions made by the authors without looking carefully at the results that underpin the conclusions. Occasionally there are instances where the conclusions in a paper are not well supported by the results presented, or where even though one treatment has been found more effective than another, the size of the gain is so slight that the results have little importance for patient care. Although researchers attempt to present an impartial view of their results, there can be a natural desire to emphasise positive aspects of the findings and minimise any potential negatives.

In this book we discuss many concepts that are useful in helping us form our own evaluation of the evidence presented in research papers. These range from the way the study is designed and the measures used, through to the meaning of the statistical results. Three aspects that are fundamental to interpreting research results are:

(1) The *size* of the effect of a treatment (or exposure). Is the effect large enough to be clinically important?
(2) Do the observed results represent a real effect, or are they likely to be a *chance finding*?
(3) Research results are always based on a *sample* of people (or objects), would we see similar results if we took another sample?

The definition of the outcome measure chosen to demonstrate the effect of a treatment (or exposure) is central to the consideration of these issues. All research studies involve measuring **outcome**. If our aim is to determine whether to use a new treatment or not, it is the effect of the treatment on a specified outcome measure that is examined. Similarly, to identify risk factors or causes of oral disease, it is the effect of the exposure of interest on the specified disease (the outcome measure) that is reported. In medicine, some outcome measures are easy to understand and have a clear clinical relevance, for example, whether the patient survives or dies, or whether the patient suffers a heart attack or not. Statins are drugs that reduce cholesterol levels and there is a large body of research evidence showing that people given statins are less likely to have a heart attack than those who are not. We can thus see a clear impact of statins on health by using the outcome measure 'heart attack or no heart attack'. Not all outcome measures in medicine and dentistry are as straightforward as this. We always need to consider whether the measure used in a particular study is both meaningful and appropriate for addressing the original question that prompted us to search for information.

Outcomes can be described as **true** or **surrogate** endpoints. True endpoints are those that have a clear and direct clinical relevance to patients[6,7]. In medicine, death is a true endpoint, as is suffering a stroke. In dentistry, the main true endpoints are pain, tooth loss, aesthetics and quality of life related to oral health, all of which are tangible to the patient. Caries status can be determined by counting the number of decayed, missing or filled teeth (DMFT). DMFT is therefore a true endpoint. Surrogate endpoints are measures that do not have an obvious impact that patients can identify easily. Periodontitis, for example, can be assessed in several ways, including measuring pocket depth or attachment level. Although simple to measure and objective, such surrogate outcomes are not always tangible to the patient. What really matters to a patient is whether teeth are lost or there is pain. A 2-mm loss of attachment does not necessarily mean that the tooth will be lost or that the patient will suffer pain.

A surrogate outcome is usually assumed to be a precursor to the true outcome. For example, if a 2-mm loss of attachment almost always leads to the loss of the tooth, pocket depth would be a good surrogate for tooth loss. Surrogate outcomes are generally objective measures that can be assessed in the short term. In treatment trials of periodontitis, changes in pocket depth or attachment level can be seen sooner than tooth loss, therefore decisions about whether to use a new treatment or not can be made earlier if the surrogate outcome is used. The assumption is that a change in the surrogate outcome measure now would produce a change in a more clinically important outcome, such as tooth loss, later on.

The evidence for routine scaling and polishing is an example in dentistry where a mixture of true and surrogate outcome measures have been used to determine whether this procedure is effective or not. Plaque, calculus, pocket depth, attachment change and bacteriological assessments are easily defined surrogates but are relevant only if they relate closely to outcomes that matter to the patient, such as tooth loss or bleeding. These outcomes are more clinically relevant, but the evidence on how much they are affected by routine scaling and polishing is scanty. Because most research in this area has used surrogate outcomes, no conclusions, at present, can be made about the effectiveness of scaling and polishing[8].

Surrogate outcome measures are used because they provide objective information quickly, and this is often a useful first step. But, there is sometimes a danger that the endpoint of clinical relevance to the patient is not investigated thoroughly and it can be hard to arrive at firm conclusions when the evidence is based solely on surrogate measures.

(4) Act on the evidence

The information obtained from assessing the evidence should then be considered in relation to the question that prompted you to undertake the search. Going back to the scenario of the woman with arthritis who has asked about the effectiveness of electric versus manual toothbrushes (see Scenario 1), there is much evidence comparing the two methods in healthy adults. Does evidence exist comparing the two in people who lack manual dexterity? If not, how far is the evidence on healthy adults likely to be relevant in this situation?

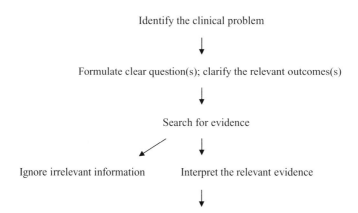

Figure 1.1 The main steps in evidence-based dentistry.

Summary

The practice of evidence-based dentistry is relatively straightforward but requires an ordered approach. The five steps are summarised in Figure 1.1.

Dentists have to elicit, sift and decide how to best use information gathered from patients, the literature, colleagues and experts in the field. Some signs and symptoms may be unexplainable, some may be difficult to treat or the patient may simply wish to discuss a treatment plan that has been recommended, but about which they are uncertain.

Therefore, it is essential to use a systematic approach when practising evidence-based dentistry. Understanding methodology makes the process easier and approaching the problem logically results in an informed decision about the best way forward. Practising evidence-based dentistry enhances patient safety and well being.

REFERENCES

1. *Adult Dental Health Survey: Oral Health in the United Kingdom 1998*. London: The Stationery Office, 2000.
2. NHS Dental Practice Board. http://www.dpb.nhs.uk/gds/latest_data.shtml (accessed in September 2005).
3. Audit Commission. *Dentistry: Primary Dental Care Services in England and Wales*, 2002 (also available at: http://www.audit-commission.gov.uk/reports/ACREPORT.asp?CatID=english%5EHEALTH&ProdID=2D847593-050A-427d-B31B-C0A4683939AA/Report_Dentistry. pdf).
4. *UK Dental Care – Market Sector Report 2003*. London: Laing & Buisson, 2003 (available at: http://www.laingbuisson.co.uk/DentistsIncome.htm).

5. American Dental Association website: http://www.ada.org/prof/resources/topics/evidencebased.asp.

6. Bader, J.D. and Ismail, A.I. A primer on outcomes in dentistry. *J Public Health Dent* 1999;**59**(3):131–135.

7. Hujoel, P.P. Endpoints in periodontal trials: the need for an evidence-based research approach. *Periodontol 2000* 2004;**36**:196–204.

8. Beirne, P., Forgie, A., Worthington, H.V. and Clarkson, J.E. Routine scale and polish for periodontal health in adults. Cochrane Review. *Cochrane Library*. Issue 1, 2005. Chichester: John Wiley.

Counting people: understanding percentages and proportions

In this chapter we present an example of the simplest type of research study. This involves taking a sample of people and counting how many of them have a certain characteristic that we are interested in. Such research is said to be descriptive. It is rarely useful in making assessments of the effectiveness of treatments or determining causes of disease.

Throughout the chapter, the discussion refers to the paper reproduced on pp. 25–30.

Reference: Underwood, B. and Fox, K. A survey of alcohol and drug use among UK based dental undergraduates. *Br Dent J* 2000; **189**: 314–317.

The numbers in the margins of the paper allow you to cross-reference between the relevant section of the paper and the discussion in this chapter (for example, *paragraph 5* is the first section of the Methods section in the paper). You should read the paper first before reading the rest of this chapter.

WHAT IS THE AIM OF THE STUDY?

Although the aim is usually stated in the title or at the beginning of the abstract, it is worthwhile clarifying in your own mind exactly what the purpose of the study is. In the article reproduced at the end of this chapter the aim is not stated in the abstract, but it is clear from the title of the paper. The abstract states that the aim is to investigate the prevalence of alcohol and recreational drug use, but it does not specify exactly in whom. From the title of the paper, it is likely that the aim is to quantify these habits in *all* dental undergraduates in UK universities in 1998 (the year when the study was done). The word 'all', although not explicitly stated in the paper, is important because it highlights the fact that we are not just interested in the habits of the dental students in this single dental school but wish to be able to make statements about all dental students in the UK in 1998.

The aim of the study can thus be stated as: To describe the proportions of dental undergraduates who smoke, who drink and who take recreational drugs in UK universities in 1998.

To quantify any characteristic of a group of people we have to decide on an appropriate measurement to express that characteristic. Here we count the number of people in a sample who have a particular characteristic, for example smoking habit (the outcome measure is, therefore, whether the student is a smoker or a non-smoker). Other characteristics of interest were alcohol use and drug use.

HOW WAS THE STUDY CONDUCTED?

The study is an example of a **prevalence study**, also called **cross-sectional study**. It is one of the simplest forms of research and is usually carried out using a **survey**. A survey involves asking people about their attributes, habits or opinions, either during a telephone or face-to-face interview with the researcher or via a postal questionnaire. The authors describe how their survey was done in *paragraphs 5–7*. Briefly, all dental undergraduates at one university were given a short questionnaire either at the start of lectures or by email during a 2-week period, and they were asked to place their completed form in a sealed box.

Another way of trying to investigate the habits of smoking, drinking and recreational drug use would be to take a **random sample** of students from all dental schools in the UK. To do this we first need a **sampling frame**. Here, this could be a list of all the students at all the dental schools. A **simple random sample** is one where every individual in the sampling frame has an equal chance of being included in the sample (computers can easily generate such lists). Because everyone has the same chance of being included in a random sample, it is likely to be representative of the whole population of interest. This means that the distribution of characteristics that could affect what we are measuring is likely to be similar in the sample and in the whole population, i.e. all dental undergraduates in the UK. We are unlikely to get particular characteristics over- or under-represented in a random sample.

The aim of a survey is to quantify specified characteristics of a defined group of people. This is achieved by estimating the **prevalence** – the number of people with the characteristic at a particular point in time, expressed as a percentage or proportion of the population of interest at the same time. Here, the aim was to quantify the prevalence of cigarette smoking, alcohol and drug use in dental students. Other examples of prevalence studies could be determining the percentage of the elderly population in the UK who are dentate or the percentage of patients on a dentist's list who visited the surgery in the last year. Such studies can usually be undertaken relatively quickly because they provide information at a single point in time. They can also be repeated over time to identify trends: for example, if the study by Underwood and Fox were repeated each year for 5 years we could see if there were changes in alcohol and drug use in dental students over that time period.

> **Box 2.1**
>
> **Prevalence** of a disease (or attribute): the proportion of people with the disease (or attribute) measured at one point in time.
>
> **Incidence rate**: the proportion of people who are new cases of the disease (or attribute) within a specified period of time.

The words **prevalence** and **incidence** are sometimes used as though they were interchangeable; they mean different things. The **incidence rate** for a disease refers to the number of *new* cases of the disease that occur during a specified *length of time* (expressed as a proportion of the number of people sampled). The **prevalence** of disease (or attribute) is the proportion of people who have the disease at *one point in time* (Box 2.1). For example, in this study the proportion of dental students who are current smokers is called the prevalence of smoking. If students had been asked whether they had taken up smoking for the first time in the previous year, then the proportion that said 'Yes' would be the incidence rate of smoking in 1 year.

WHAT ARE THE MAIN RESULTS?

It is not always clear where to find the important results in a paper. Although the main results are usually given in the abstract, they can also be found within the body of the text. Sometimes so many results are presented that it is difficult to identify those which are important. Occasionally the conclusions in the paper are not adequately supported by the results. When interpreting results it is useful to first identify the ones which relate specifically to the aim of the study.

Current cigarette smoking

Paragraph 12 shows some of the results on smoking. For example, the prevalence of smoking in fourth and fifth year males is 21%, that is, of all the males in Years 4–5, 21% currently smoke.

Sometimes it is worth generating tables yourself using data given in the paper, as this may simplify the results you are interested in and make them easier to interpret. Table 2.1 was not given in the paper but can be derived from the results given in the text (*paragraph 12*) and the number of male and female students in the study from *Table 2* (column labelled 'n') of the paper.

The first result to look at is the overall percentage of students who smoke (the last row of Table 2.1). The overall prevalence of smoking is estimated by observing how many smokers there were out of the total number of students. In Table 2.1, 198 students responded to the survey, of whom 15 said that they smoked. The prevalence is thus 15/198 or 8% or 8 in every 100 students. It can also be represented as a proportion,

Table 2.1 The prevalence of smoking according to gender and year of study.

Gender	Year of study	Prevalence	Number of smokers/total number of students
Males	Years 1–3	4%	2/53
	Years 4–5	21%	7/34
	All years	*10%*	*9/87*
Females	Years 1–3	1%	1/73
	Years 4–5	13%	5/38
	All years	*5%*	*6/111*
All students	Years 1–3	2%	3/126
	Years 4–5	17%	12/72
All students	All years	8%	15/198

0.08. When we look at particular subgroups of people, we divide by the number of people in the subgroup, not by the number in the whole sample. For example, there were 87 males in the study and nine of them smoked: a prevalence of 10% among males (9/87).

Alcohol

Alcohol consumption was described using two different outcome measures, total intake over the last week and binge drinking during a typical session. These characterise different aspects of the students' alcohol habits.

The results on alcohol use are summarised in *paragraphs 13–15*, *Figure 1* and *Table 1* of the paper. The figure is a **bar chart** that illustrates, at a glance, the distribution of alcohol intake according to gender and year of study. Such figures are common in clinical research papers and they avoid having cumbersome sections of text or tables that are filled with many numbers. For example, it is easy to see that the percentage of males in Years 1–3 who have sensible levels of alcohol intake (0–21 units per week, shown in the lower section of each bar) is about 50% (prevalence of 50%) and that this is greater than in Years 4–5. *Table 1* provides other information on alcohol use – whereas *Figure 1* summarises intake during the week before completing the questionnaire, *Table 1* describes binge drinking, that is, alcohol intake during a single session. The prevalence of binge drinking among students who consume alcohol is high: 55.6% in males and 58.5% in females.

Recreational drug use

Several recreational drugs were looked at and the prevalence of each of these is reported in the text (*paragraphs 16–20*) and *Table 2*. Because cannabis was the most commonly used drug, the authors concentrated on this and provided data according to gender and year of study. Overall, the prevalence of cannabis use at any time is about 55% (calculated by subtracting 44.9% from 100% in *Table 2*).

Comparisons between groups

Once the overall prevalence for each habit has been obtained, we can see whether prevalence differs between groups of people, for example, by gender or year of study. In discussing differences between groups prevalence can be referred to as a **risk**. For example, the prevalence of students who smoke in Years 4–5 is 17% and this can also be described as 'the risk of being a smoker in Years 4–5 is 17%'. It is clear that the risk of smoking in Years 4–5 (17%) is greater than that in Years 1–3 (2%) (Table 2.1). There are two ways of describing this comparison numerically. We could subtract one risk from the other, called the **absolute risk difference**, 17% – 2%, which means that there are 15% additional smokers in Years 4–5 than in Years 1–3. Alternatively, we could take the ratio of the two risks, which tells us how many times more likely the 4- and 5-year students are to smoke than those in Years 1–3. They are about 8 times more likely to smoke (17% ÷ 2%). This estimate of '8 times more likely' is called a **relative risk** (or **risk ratio**); it is a common measure used when assessing causes, prevention and treatment of death or disease.

Risk difference and relative risk are both valid ways of presenting the information: they each tell us something useful. Describing the absolute difference as 15% tells us that if we take 100 students from Years 1–3 and 100 from Years 4–5, we could expect to find 15 more smokers in Years 4–5 than in Years 1–3. The relative risk tells us that students in Years 4–5 are 8 times more likely to smoke than students in Years 1–3, but we cannot tell from this *how many additional* students smoke. For example, 8 times more likely could equally well describe 80 students in Years 4–5 compared with 10 students in Years 1–3 (a difference of 70 people) as it could 16 students in Years 4–5 and 2 in Years 1–3 (a difference of 14 people). Both examples are associated with the same relative risk but the number of additional students who smoke (risk difference) is very dissimilar (Box 2.2). More discussion of relative risks and risk difference, and their interpretation is found in Chapters 4–6 and 8.

We can also compare the prevalence of binge drinking between males and females (among students who consume alcohol). Table 2.2 shows the results in *Table 1* from the paper in a different format. Overall the prevalence of binge drinking is similar in male and female students (56% males, 58% females), but there is a difference according to

---

Box 2.2

Definition	Example (risk of being current smoker)
Risk in Group A = p_A Risk in Group B = p_B	Risk in students in Years 4–5 = 0.17 (= 17%) Risk in students in Years 1–3 = 0.02 (= 2%)
Absolute risk difference = $p_A - p_B$ Relative risk = p_A/p_B (in Group A compared with Group B)	Absolute risk difference = 0.17 – 0.02 = 0.15 (= 15%) Relative risk = 0.17/0.2 = 8.5 (in Group A compared with Group B)

Table 2.2 Prevalence of binge drinking according to gender and year of study.

Year of study	Prevalence of binge drinking (%)	
	Males	**Females**
1–3 (R1)	45	69
4–5 (R2)	70	40
All	56	58
Relative risk (R2/R1)	1.6	0.6

year of study. Male students tend to binge drink later on in their studies (they are 1.6 times as likely to binge drink in Years 4–5 as Years 1–3), while female students tend to do this earlier on (they are 0.6 times as likely to binge drink in Years 4–5 as Years 1–3). We could try to ascertain the reasons for this apparent difference in habits.

THE IMPLICATIONS OF CONDUCTING A STUDY BASED ON A SAMPLE OF PEOPLE

What we are really interested in is the prevalence of these habits, for example, cannabis use in the whole population of UK dental students in 1998. At the time of the study there were 13 dental schools in the UK with a total of about 5000 students. However, we have the results from only one dental school. Is it possible to extrapolate the results to all UK dental students in 1998? For example, about 55% of students in the study had tried or were current users of cannabis (*paragraph 19*). If we had been able to conduct the survey on every single dental student in the UK (that is, all 5000) would we still see a prevalence of 55%? Although it is unlikely to be 55% exactly, we might expect that it would not be far off.

The estimate based on all dental students is referred to as the **true** or **population** prevalence. It is something we can rarely obtain in research since it is usually impossible to conduct a survey on every single individual of interest. The concept of a true (or population) value is central to interpreting research and forms one of the core themes throughout this book. How can the true prevalence be estimated when we only have a sample of people?

When a sample is surveyed instead of the whole population there will always be some uncertainty over how far our observed estimate is from the true prevalence. This uncertainty can be quantified by the **standard error**. If a study was based on the whole population, we would have the true prevalence and there would be no uncertainty; the standard error would be 0. If we took several different samples of the same size they would all give slightly different estimates of prevalence. The standard error measures how much we expect sample prevalences to spread out around the true prevalence. The amount of spread that we expect depends on the size of the

Box 2.3

Standard error of a prevalence is a measure of the uncertainty associated with trying to estimate the true prevalence when we only have a sample.
   If observed prevalence $= p$, and sample size $= n$ then

$$\text{Standard error} = \sqrt{\frac{p(1 - p)}{n}}$$

Example: a prevalence of 55% based on 198 students $p = 0.55, n = 198$
Standard error $= \sqrt{0.55 \times (1 - 0.55)/198} = 0.0354$

sample. If our sample size is very large, for example we survey 4000 dental students, we are likely to get a good estimate that is close to the true prevalence. If our sample size is small, for example we only sample ten students, then we could get an estimate that is very different from the true prevalence. The formula used to calculate the standard error takes sample size into account (Box 2.3). The n on the bottom of the equation means that as the sample size gets larger the standard error will get smaller. One of the most powerful uses of a standard error is that it enables us to calculate a **confidence interval** (Box 2.4).

A **confidence interval for the (true) prevalence** is a range within which we expect the true prevalence to lie. In the study of 198 students, the prevalence of ever-cannabis use was 55%. But we know that in the population of all dental UK undergraduates the true value may be greater or smaller than this. The **95% confidence interval** for the prevalence of cannabis use is 48% to 62%. We interpret this information by saying that using the results from the study, the best estimate of the true prevalence is 55%, but we are 95% sure (or confident) that the true prevalence lies somewhere between

Box 2.4

Calculating a 95% confidence interval (CI) for a prevalence
   Lower limit of CI $=$ observed prevalence $- 1.96 \times$ standard error of prevalence
   Upper limit of CI $=$ observed prevalence $+ 1.96 \times$ standard error of prevalence

Example: a prevalence of 55% based on 198 students

$$p = 0.55, n = 198$$
$$\text{Standard error} = 0.0354$$
$$95\% \text{ CI} = 0.55 \pm 1.96 \times 0.0354 = 0.48 \text{ to } 0.62 \text{ (or 48 to 62\%)}$$

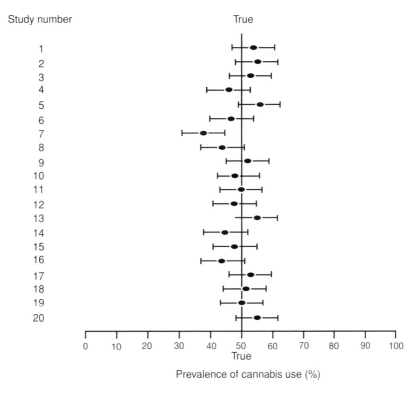

Figure 2.1 The prevalence of cannabis use among UK dental undergraduates in the study by Underwood and Fox (2000) and 19 hypothetical studies of the same size. Each dot represents the estimate of prevalence, and the ends of the line are the lower and upper limits of the 95% confidence interval. The vertical line (at 50%) is assumed to be the true prevalence (the one based on all UK undergraduates).

48% and 62%[*]. So even the most conservative estimate of cannabis use is that about half (48%) of all dental students had tried or currently use it. It could also be that as many as 62% of students had tried it or use it.

Why is '95%' used as the level of confidence? This is the most commonly used level in research and was chosen many decades ago. It is somewhat arbitrary but judged to be a sufficiently high level of confidence. There is nothing special or scientific about '95%', and you sometimes see 90% or even 99% confidence intervals. The multiplier '1.96' is associated with using a 95% range.

By definition a 95% confidence interval means that we would expect to miss the true prevalence 5% of the time. Figure 2.1 illustrates the concept of confidence intervals using the one from the published study (study number 1) and results from

[*] The more exact definition is that we expect 95% of such intervals to contain the true prevalence. Although this seems like a subtle distinction, it is often easier to interpret confidence intervals using our original definition and little is lost by this.

Box 2.5

95% confidence interval for a prevalence: this is a range of plausible values for the **true** prevalence based on our data. It is a range within which the true value is expected to lie with high degree of certainty. If confidence intervals were calculated from many different studies of the same size, we expect about 95% of them would contain the true prevalence, and 5% would not

---

19 hypothetical studies, all based on the same number of students as the published one (that is, 198 students). In the figure we assume that we know the true prevalence and it is 50% (that is, the prevalence in all 5000 students in the UK had we been able to undertake such a survey). Each of the 20 studies gives an estimate of the true prevalence. Some studies will give an estimate above 50%, others below 50% and occasionally 50% exactly, but all have confidence intervals that include 50% except one study (number 7). Because 95% confidence intervals are used, 5% of confidence intervals (1 in every 20 studies) are expected *not* to include the true prevalence (Box 2.5).

The width of the confidence interval for the true prevalence will depend on the number of individuals in the study. This is illustrated in Figure 2.2, which gives 95% confidence intervals for studies based on 50 to 4000 students. If it had been possible to survey all 5000 dental students in the UK in 1998 we would know the true prevalence and there would be no confidence interval. The larger the study (and the closer we get to our 5000 students) the more confident we become in believing that our observed estimate is equal or very close to the true prevalence. The 95% confidence interval range becomes narrower, the lower and upper limits are closer to the observed prevalence in the study. If fewer students are included, we get further away from the 5000 and we become less certain that our observed estimate is close to the true prevalence. The confidence interval range becomes wider. It is difficult to draw firm conclusions from research when the confidence intervals are wide (for example 5% to 85%) since the likely true prevalence could be very low or very high (Box 2.6).

In using a sample to estimate the true prevalence we need to assume that the characteristics of the sample (students in the one dental school) are similar to those of all UK students. Can the results from the single study by Underwood and Fox be extrapolated to the whole population of dental students? We should consider whether the students may or may not be representative of all UK students. The

---

Box 2.6

LARGE study $\longrightarrow$ small standard error $\longrightarrow$ narrow confidence interval
small study $\longrightarrow$ LARGE standard error $\longrightarrow$ WIDE confidence interval

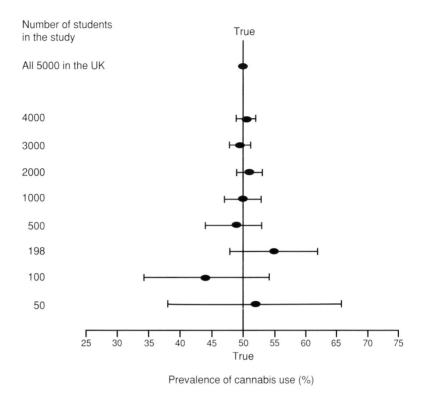

Figure 2.2 Estimates of the prevalence of cannabis use among UK dental undergraduates in the study by Underwood and Fox (2000), third study from the bottom (n = 198) and seven hypothetical studies of different sizes. Each dot represents the estimate of prevalence, and the ends of the line are the lower and upper limits of the 95% confidence interval. The vertical line (at 50%) is assumed to be the true prevalence (the one based on all UK undergraduates).

authors of the paper thought that their students might have similar habits to those of students in other universities (*paragraph 24*), although they were not a random sample from all UK schools. However, the students came from only one school in a single geographical location, so they may not be representative of all dental students.

HOW GOOD IS THE EVIDENCE?

Determining how good the evidence is will depend on how the study was conducted, who is in the sample and how the results were analysed. There is no such thing as the perfect study, and researchers often look back and with hindsight see ways of improving their study after it has ended. We have already examined the main results, so the purpose of this section is to see whether there are any features of the study that might influence our interpretation of the results, as well as any strengths of the study that help support the conclusions.

> **Box 2.7**
>
> **Bias**: any influence which means that the result from a study (for example prevalence or incidence) is systematically overestimated or underestimated compared with the true underlying value.
>
> Bias can arise from the way people respond to a study, characteristics of these people or the way researchers have conducted the study

Are there any biases?

We need to consider if there were any **biases** that may have affected the results. A bias is some factor or characteristic of the study, of people in the study or of the way the researchers have designed the study, that shifts the results in a particular direction such that the observed results are an overestimate or underestimate of the true underlying value (Box 2.7). Biases should not be confused with **random** (or **chance**) **variation** which only reflect natural differences between people. Here we give some examples of possible biases; further examples will be discussed in later chapters. One way to determine if and how biases can affect the results is to imagine yourself to be either the respondent or the researcher and then ask yourself, 'How can I *adversely* affect the results, so they do not reflect what is really going on?'.

How could the respondents bias the results?

Respondents can bias results in two ways: those who do not respond at all may be different from responders, and those who do respond may give incorrect information. Some examples of these are as follows.

- **Response bias**. Certain subgroups of students may be less likely to respond at all to the questionnaire. For example, those from cultural backgrounds where alcohol and drugs are prohibited may not want to be included in this study. If such students are less likely to drink or use drugs, the estimates of prevalence observed would be higher than the true prevalence. Similarly, students who have severe alcoholic or drug use problems may be less likely to respond and this would result in underestimates of the prevalence of alcohol and drug use.
- **Misreporting bias**. Some responders may give incorrect information. A subject could over or under-report their habits. For example, current cigarette smokers may say that they have never smoked, or smokers of 40 cigarettes per day may say that they only smoke 10 cigarettes per day. Alternatively, there could be non-smokers who say they smoke.

How misreporting produces a bias:
Table 2.3 illustrates how bias can arise and affect the results of a study. If one group of people are more likely to misreport their habits than the other group the observed

Table 2.3 Hypothetical study of 100 dental students, where their true smoking status is known and compared with their reported smoking status. It is assumed that 10 smokers lie and report themselves as non-smokers.

	Reported smoker	Reported non-smoker	Total	
True smoker	20	10	30	True prevalence is 30%
True non-smoker	0	70	70	
Total	20	80	100	
	Observed smoking prevalence is 20%			

results would not measure the true prevalence accurately. For example, if 10 smokers misreport as non-smokers we would estimate the smoking prevalence to be 20% when in fact it is 30%.

Misreporting in this way would have the effect of *underestimating* the true prevalence of smoking in dental students. This illustrates the fact that bias can only arise when there is *a shift in one direction*. If there were an equal number of non-smokers who misreport as smokers, the estimate of the prevalence would not be biased. However, we know that non-smokers are highly unlikely to say that they smoke. So there will be more smokers who misreport, and therefore surveys tend to under-report the prevalence of smoking.

How could the research design bias the results?

- **Observer bias**. Because the questionnaire was completed by the student and not during a face-to-face interview with one of the researchers, it is not possible for the attitude of the researcher to bias the responses; there is no observer bias.
- **Investigator bias**. The questionnaire could have been phrased in such a way that the responses fulfil the expectations of the researchers. For example, there may be questions that encourage students who drink alcohol to report that their use is greater than it really is. We would need to see the questionnaire for evidence of this.

Strengths and limitations

When reading a paper we should consider the extent to which the study design and analysis of the data allow the aim of the study to be addressed. This can be done by listing the main strengths and limitations of the particular study, and from these making a judgement on the validity of the results and whether they are generally applicable or not. Below are some of the strengths and limitations of this paper. Similar considerations will apply to any other study. You may find it useful to write your own list before reading the one below.

Strengths

(1) The survey included students from all 5 years of study so it is possible to observe whether the habits differ according to year of study (*paragraph 5*). If, for example, only first year students were included, we could not be sure that their habits would be similar to students in other years, particularly fifth (final) year students.

(2) The questionnaire was anonymous (*paragraph 8*). Because the students cannot be identified they are more likely to respond and less likely to lie, especially over the use of illegal substances such as cannabis.

(3) Students were asked to report how much alcohol they had consumed in the week previous to completing the questionnaire (*paragraph 14*), which they are likely to remember more accurately than if they tried trying to estimate it over a longer period.

(4) The questionnaire was piloted on 25 medical students (*paragraph 7*). This was to ensure that the questions were phrased clearly.

(5) There was a reasonably high **response rate**. Here, the response rate is the percentage of students who sent the questionnaire back to the researchers. From a total of 264 dental students (*paragraph 5*), 200 replied (*paragraph 9*); a response rate of 76%. There is no generally agreed acceptable response rate but clearly 90% is very good and 10% is poor. We do not, however, know if all the questions had been completed by all the responders. In other studies, response rate could be defined as the proportion of people who respond and have completed a sufficient number of questions. Are the characteristics of the 24% non-responders likely to be very different from those of the responders? Since few surveys have a 100% response rate it is worth considering whether the actual response rate from a particular study was sufficiently high and to see if the researchers made some attempt to ascertain the characteristics of the non-responders. Sometimes researchers will contact a random sample of non-responders in order to determine their characteristics and perhaps ask their reasons for not responding.

(6) Smoking habits before and after entry to the dental school were ascertained ('Subjects and methods' in the abstract). This allowed a comparison of the proportion who smoked at these two times (*paragraph 23*).

Limitations

(1) Although the title of the paper implies we are interested in the habits of dental students in all dental schools in the UK in 1998, only one dental school was included in the study (*paragraph 5*). To be able to apply the results to all UK dental students we would have to assume that the characteristics of the students in this particular school were similar to those in all UK dental schools. If students tended to come from anywhere in the country this assumption could be true. On the other hand, access to cannabis and alcohol may have varied from school to school. It is stated in the Discussion (*paragraph 25*) that this dental school had a high proportion of

students from ethnic minorities, who might have a lower consumption of alcohol, illegal drugs and cigarettes. If this assumption was correct then the estimates of prevalence from this study would be underestimates compared with those from other schools.

(2) The study was done in 1998 (*paragraph 7*) and not published until 2000, and the habits of students may have changed since then. Are the results applicable to students today or have they changed substantially?

(3) The measurement of cigarette, alcohol, and cannabis consumption relies on self-reporting, therefore the accuracy of this depends on accurate recall and students telling the truth. Both are common concerns when people complete questionnaires about their characteristics and lifestyles. People find it difficult to remember details about their life many years ago and some may lie when faced with questions of a sensitive nature (for example sexual habits). It is useful, therefore, to look carefully at what is being asked and how likely it is that people will be unable to recall information accurately or lie. The researchers attempted to determine the extent of misreporting and thought that the students did report their habits accurately (*paragraph 25*).

(4) We do not know if any of the characteristics of the 24% of students who did not respond to the questionnaire differed from those who did respond.

Consistency with other studies

We could compare the results with those from other surveys conducted at a similar time. For example, the General Household Survey provides the prevalence of various lifestyle habits in the general adult population in Great Britain. In the age group 20–24 years the prevalence was 42% in males and 39% in females, compared with 10% and 5% in male and female dental students, found by Underwood and Fox. Dental students are therefore much less likely to smoke than people of a similar age in the general population.

WHAT DOES THE STUDY CONTRIBUTE TO DENTAL PRACTICE?

At first glance the results do not appear to impact directly on general dental practice. However, the health and habits of practising clinicians can affect the care they give their patients. Since many students drink alcohol and a high proportion had used illegal drugs, this could affect exam performance, clinical performance and have long-term health effects. Dental schools may judge that some kind of support should be provided for students. The results also raise the question of whether the excess alcohol intake and drug use continues after qualifying. It is often the case that a study that answers one research question leads to the identification of further research topics.

Key points

- Prevalence of a disease is the proportion of people who have the disease at one point in time.
- Incidence rate of a disease is the proportion of people who are new cases of the disease within a specified period of time.
- Relative risk and absolute risk difference are measures that compare proportions (or percentages) in two groups.
- Standard error of a prevalence is a measure of the uncertainty associated with trying to estimate the *true* prevalence when we only have a sample.
- A confidence interval provides a range within which the true (population) prevalence or incidence is likely to lie
- When reading a cross-sectional study consider:
  - the aim of the study
  - the sample
  - potential biases
  - strengths and limitations of the way the study was conducted and how the results were analysed
  - who the results will apply to.

Acknowledgement

We are grateful to the *British Dental Journal* and Ben Underwood for kindly giving permission to reproduce the article in this chapter.

Exercise

Consider the following questions in relation to the paper by Underwood and Fox (2000):
(1) What is the overall prevalence of current regular users of cannabis in this study? From this estimate how many students in the study responded that they were current regular users?
(2) Does the prevalence of current regular cannabis use vary according to gender and year of study?
(3) What is the relative risk of being a current smoker if you were a previous smoker compared with if you were not a previous smoker? Interpret the relative risk.
(4) It is generally well known that people who smoke are more likely to drink alcohol. If dental students who smoke heavily are less likely to respond to the questionnaire, what effect would this have on the estimated prevalence of alcohol drinking?

Answers on pp. 209

A survey of alcohol and drug use among UK based dental undergraduates

B. Underwood[1] and K. Fox

Objective This study was designed to investigate the prevalence of alcohol and drug use.
Design Anonymous self-report questionnaire
Setting A UK dental school in May 1998
Subjects and methods 1st–5th year dental undergraduates (n = 264) were questioned on their use of alcohol and tobacco, cannabis and other illicit drugs whilst at dental school, and before entry.
Results Eighty two per cent of male and 90% of female undergraduates reported drinking alcohol. Of those drinking, 63% of males and 42% of females drank in excess of sensible weekly limits (14 units for females, 21 units for males), with 56% of males and 58.5% of females 'binge drinking'. Regular tobacco smoking (10 or more cigarettes a day) was found to have a statistically significant association with year of study, 4th-5th year undergraduates being eight times more likely to regularly smoke than their junior colleagues. Fifty five per cent of undergraduates reported cannabis use at least once or twice since starting dental school, with 8% of males and 6% of females reporting current regular use at least once a week.
Conclusion Dental undergraduates are drinking above sensible weekly limits of alcohol, binge drinking and indulging in illicit drug use. Dental Schools should designate a teacher responsible for education of undergraduates regarding alcohol and substance abuse.

[1]*Red Lea Dental Practice, Market Place, Easingwold North Yorkshire, YO61 3AD*
Correspondence to: B. Underwood
REFEREED PAPER
Received 18.10.00; Accepted 18.07.00
© *British Dental Journal* 2000; 189: 314–417

Alcohol and drug use among UK school children and university students is increasing.[1,2,3,4,5] A recent nation-wide survey[6] of second-year university students from a range of faculties found many consuming alcohol above sensible limits[7,8,9] and using cannabis and other illicit drugs. Binge drinking[10] has also been widely reported among students,[11,12,13] with established associated health risks and connections with anti-social behaviour.

Surveys of medical students' alcohol[11,12] and drug use[13,14] have shown similar high levels to their

RESEARCH
<u>law</u> and <u>ethics</u>

non-medical counterparts. Alarmingly, medical students constitute a group who will exert an influence disproportionate to its numbers on future social and economic health in the UK,[13] a fact also applicable to dental under-graduates.

3 The Dental Health Support Programme, formerly known as the Sick Dentists' Scheme, was founded in 1986 with the aim of supporting qualified dentists with alcohol and drug addictions and has to date helped over 500 UK dentists;[15] the high incidence giving cause for concern in the profession. This concern is now being felt at the undergraduate level, with the new GDC guidelines stating:

> *Behaviour reflecting adversely on the profession, such as dishonesty, indecency or violence; convictions in a court of law; or problems related to alcohol or drugs, during the time as an undergraduate dental student could lead to the first application for registration being referred to the President. It could easily be taken into consideration later if the Council had cause to consider the conduct of a registered dentist.*[16]

4 Prior to this study, no significant information existed on the prevalence of alcohol and drug use among UK dental undergraduates. This information is needed before the current concerns can be addressed, and will provide a basis for future research and education.

Method

5 A survey was conducted at one UK dental school of all undergraduates studying in years 1 to 5 (n = 264). A self-report questionnaire was distributed, by the organiser, to 2nd, 3rd and 4th year students before scheduled lectures. Absentees, 1st and 5th year students were contacted via internal mail.

6 The questionnaire consisted of 4 sides of A4 text on a folded A3 sheet, the cover page acting as a participant information sheet. Questions were asked in closed ended format in standard English making them easily answered, scored and coded (for analysis by computer). The length of the questionnaire was kept as short as feasible allowing completion in less than 5 minutes. Participants were provided with a free pen to act as an incentive and increase anonymity. Return of completed questionnaires was via a self-seal envelope labelled with the organiser's name. In addition the label gave the location of a sealed respondents' box.

7 The questionnaire was administered over a 2 week period from the 25th May 1998 to the 5th June 1998, avoiding Dental Student Society social events or examination periods, which may not have represented an average week. Prior to distribution, the questionnaire was piloted on 25 medical students, 5 from each year. This highlighted only minor problems that were then corrected before full-scale administration.

8 Anonymity of participants was essential and, therefore, no name or ethnic group was requested, also no individual questionnaire or year group responses were reported. It was stressed that completion of the questionnaire was voluntary, with no obligation to respond. Confidentiality was strictly maintained with all completed questionnaires being seen exclusively by the survey organiser.

9 The response rate was high, with 200 undergraduates completing the questionnaire, one respondent who omitted their gender and year was not included in the study.

Ethical approval

10 Ethical approval was granted by the local research ethics committee. Consent for the questionnaire to be distributed at the Dental School was given by the senior staff.

Statistical analysis

11 Statistical analysis was carried out using SPSS for Windows. Analysis using a variety of non-parametric techniques was undertaken. Results are descriptive and basically quantitative. Associations between variables were analysed by the Chi-square test and Fisher's exact test.

Results

Tobacco

12 Regular tobacco use (10 or more cigarettes per day) was most highly reported among 4th and 5th year males with 21% currently smoking and 15% smoking prior to becoming undergraduates. Only 4% of 1st to 3rd year males reported current regular tobacco use with 6% reporting regular use before entering dental school. Tobacco use among female undergraduates showed similar findings to their male colleagues, with 13% of 4th and 5th years regularly smoking and 1% of 1st to 3rd years, however 22% of 1st to 3rd year females reported smoking tobacco only whilst drinking.

Alcohol

13 Eighty two per cent of males and 90% of females reported drinking alcohol. Of those drinking 'sensible levels' (0–21 units per week male, 0–14 units female) were exceeded by 63% of males and 42% females. Hazardous drinking, >50 units per week for males, >35 units for females, was reported by 13% of males and 7% of females (Figure 1).

14 Figures are reported as units of alcohol consumed last week, as they were found to be consistently higher than those which the undergraduates

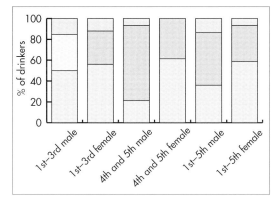

Fig. 1 Level of alcohol consumption by dental undergraduates. Green, hazardous to health level of alcohol consumption; red, increased risk; yellow, sensible level of alcohol being consumed.

Table 1 Binge drinking by dental undergraduates

Gender and Year	n	Binge drinking %
Male 1–3	42	45.2
Female 1–3	64	68.7
Male 4–5	30	70.0
Female 4–5	36	40.0
Male 1–5	73	55.6
Female 1–5	100	58.5

reported as their average number of units consumed weekly.

15 Binge drinking,[10] (defined as drinking half the recommended weekly units of alcohol in one session, i.e. at least seven units for women and 10 units for men) was reported by 56% of males and 58.5% of females with 70% of 4th and 5th year males reporting binge drinking (Table 1). Thirty per cent of those drinking alcohol overestimated their safe weekly maximum consumption (11% of males and 4% of females if Department of Health limits are used) and 71% reported their alcohol intake was less prior to becoming a dental undergraduate.

Cannabis

16 Sixty two per cent of males and 49.5% of females reported cannabis use since becoming a dental undergraduate, with 44% of males having used cannabis more than once or twice and 8% reporting current regular use (regular being defined as at least once a week). Twenty six percent of females reported having used cannabis more than once or twice whilst an undergraduate, 6% reporting current regular use.

17 Highest current regular cannabis use was reported amongst male 4th and 5th year undergraduates as 15%, with 59% reporting having used cannabis more than once or twice and 15% reporting regular cannabis use before entering dental school (Table 2). Lowest regular cannabis use was reported by male 1st–3rd years as 4%.

RESEARCH
law and ethics

Table 2 Cannabis use since becoming a dental undergraduate

Gender and year	n	Never %	once or twice %	>once or twice %	past regular user, but not in current year of study %	past regular user but not now %	current regular user %
Male 1–3	53	45.3	20.8	26.4	3.8	0.0	3.8
Female 1–3	73	54.8	26.0	9.6	4.1	1.4	4.1
Male 4–5	34	26.5	14.7	23.5	14.7	5.9	14.7
Female 4–5	38	42.1	18.4	15.8	5.3	7.9	10.5
Male 1–5	87	37.9	18.4	25.3	8.0	2.3	8.0
Female 1–5	111	50.5	23.4	11.7	4.5	3.6	6.3
Whole	198	44.9	21.2	17.7	6.1	3.0	7.1

18 **Other illicit drugs, amyl nitrate and inhalant use**
Forty five per cent of males and 34% of females reported illicit drug use other than cannabis whilst a dental undergraduate, with 40% of males and 31% of females reporting use before entry to dental school. These figures increase, when amyl nitrate and inhalants (which are not classified as illegal drugs) are included, to 48% of males and 36% of females using drugs whilst undergraduates and 45% of males and 33.5% of females having used drugs prior to entry.

19 After cannabis (55%) the next most commonly used drugs whilst a dental undergraduate were, amphetamines (16%), amyl nitrate (13%), Ecstasy and magic mushrooms (8%), LSD (5.5%), cocaine (4.5%) and inhalants (2.5%).

20 Current regular drug use other than cannabis was rarely reported, with 2.9% of 4th–5th year males using amphetamines and 1.4% of 1st–3rd year females using ecstasy at least once a month.

Associations

21 A highly statistically significant association between year of under-graduate study and regular tobacco use was found (p < 0.001), with 4th–5th year undergraduates being eight times more likely to regularly smoke tobacco than their 1st–3rd year colleagues.

22 No significant associations were found between year of under-graduate study and drinking over sensible weekly limits or regular cannabis use. There was no significant association between those who drank above sensible limits and smoked tobacco on a regular basis.

23 Those smoking regularly before entering dental school were found to be statistically significantly more likely to be a current regular tobacco smoker (p < 0.001). Of the 14 undergraduates regularly smoking before entering dental school, 9 had continued to regularly smoke, whereas only 6 undergraduates out of 184 had become regular smokers since entry to dental school.

Discussion

24 The results of this survey reflect drug and alcohol use among under-graduates at one UK dental school. However, there is little reason to suspect students at the university surveyed are unique in their experiences. Unpublished data from a recent study of 75% of all vocational dental practitioners revealed a similar level of alcohol and drug use during their times as undergraduates.

25 A high response rate was achieved, with 76% of undergraduates completing the questionnaire. Honesty of responses is difficult to access, as with all self-report surveys, but discussions with participants after the survey suggested truthful responses had been reported, with methods used to maintain anonymity being appreciated. For ethical reasons individual year's responses are not reported due to fears of a breach of anonymity. Ethnic background was not questioned. This may affect the results of the study, as there is a large group of

ethnic minority students in the dental school. It has been found in previous studies[6,13] that these groups have much lower levels of alcohol consumption, cannabis use and tobacco smoking than whites.

26 Figures quoted for sensible weekly alcohol consumption levels (14 units for women, 21 units for men) throughout this report are those recommended by the British Medical Association[7] and The Royal College of Physicians, Psychiatrists, and General Practitioners.[8] These are lower than the levels recommended by the Department of Health,[17] (21 units for women, 28 units for men) which have been criticised.[9]

27 Of those drinking alcohol, 63% of male and 42% of female under-graduates surveyed drank over sensible limits for their gender, levels similar to those reported by students in general[6] (61% males, 48% females), an obvious cause for concern. More alarming is how alcohol is consumed, with binge drinking[10] being reported by 56% of male and 58.5% of female dental undergraduates, this is double that found in university students in general (28%). Highest levels of binge drinking were reported by male 4th–5th years and female 1st–3rd years at 70% and 69% respectively. The reason for this pattern of alcohol consumption may be due to students restricting drinking during the week because of clinical commitments and then binging at weekends. Binge drinking with resultant inebriation has been associated with unprotected sexual contacts, unplanned pregnancies and sexually transmitted diseases, such as HIV.[18,19] Links between crime (especially violent crime) and heavy drinking[20,21] have been found, with drink related crime being highest among young males who have been binge drinking at weekends. It would be hard to deny the enjoyment associated with drinking alcohol. There is however, a point after which the hazards outweigh the benefits. Despite formal guidance given on professionalism within the dental course, there would still appear to be a prevalent culture of heavy drinking by undergraduates. Without further

intervention this is likely to continue with inevitable consequences.

28 Regular tobacco smoking (10 or more cigarettes per day) was found to have statistically significant associations ($p < 0.001$) with year of study, senior undergraduates of both sexes being more likely to smoke regularly than their juniors. Due to the cross sectional nature of this survey, it is not possible to say whether there is an upward progression in frequency of smoking from first through fifth year. Twenty one per cent of male and 13% of female 4th–5th years reported smoking at least 10 cigarettes a day, and 21% of female 1st–3rd years reported smoking only whilst drinking. This gives cause for concern, as these individuals will have future responsibility for the health care of the general population.

29 Regular cannabis use (weekly or more often) by dental under-graduates was found to be lower than that by students in general,[6] at 8% by males and 6% by females compared to 23% and 16%. Fifty five per cent of dental undergraduates reported cannabis use at least once or twice since coming to dental school, therefore, over half of undergraduates have used a Class B illegal drug, and in doing so risk possible criminal convictions with wider ramifications for future employment or even registration.

30 Illicit drug use, other than cannabis, (excluding amyl nitrate and inhalants, which are not illegal to use) was reported by 45% of male and 34% of female undergraduates, whilst at dental school, 40% of males and 31% of females reporting use before becoming an under-graduate. This is lower than that found in university students[6] in general at 59%, this figure does however, include amyl nitrate. Regular illicit drug use (once a month or more often), other than cannabis was rarely reported.

31 This study gives only a snapshot of the current situation, and it is not known how those surveyed will change in their habits once qualified, therefore the results of this survey should be used as a baseline. Longitudinal studies of those participating in

RESEARCH
law and ethics

this survey should be carried out yearly to monitor changes in drug and alcohol use during vocational training and beyond. It may also be advisable to survey levels of stress in future studies, as a recent BDA survey[22] found high levels of alcohol consumption by dentists was associated with raised stress levels.

In conclusion, this survey has found undergraduates at the dental school surveyed drinking above sensible weekly limits, binge drinking and indulging in illicit drug use to a degree which may damage health and future careers. The Royal College of Physicians of Edinburgh and the Medical Council on Alcoholism, recommend medical schools designate a teacher responsible for education of students about alcohol and substance abuse and for monitoring the impact of such information.[23] This advice is also applicable to Dental Schools.

The authors gratefully acknowledge all undergraduates who took part in this study, Dr B. Scaife for statistical support and Dr P. N. Nixon for advice on questionnaire design.

1 Plant M, Plant M. *Risk-takers: alcohol, drugs, sex and youth.* London: Tavistock/Routledge, 1992.

2 Balding J. *Young people in 1993* Exeter Schools Health Education Unit; University of Exeter, 1994.

3 Wright J D, Pearl L. Knowledge and experience of young people regarding drug misuse, 1969–94. *Br Med J* 1995; 310: 20–24.

4 Calman K. On the state of public health. *Health Trends* 1995; 27:71–75.

5 Royal College of Physicians. Alcohol and the young. *J R Coll Phys London* 1995; 29: 470–74.

6 Webb E, Ashton C H, Kelly P, Kamali F. Alcohol and drug use in UK university students. *The Lancet* 1996; 348: 922–25.

7 British Medical Association. *Alcohol: guidelines on sensible drinking.* London BMA, 1995.

8 Royal College of Physicians, Psychiatrists, and General Practitioners. *Alcohol and the heart in perspective: sensible limits reaffirmed.* London: Royal Colleges, 1995.

9 Edward G. Sensible drinking: doctors should stick with the independent medical advice. *Br Med J* 1996; 312: 1.

10 Moore L, Smith C, Catford J. Binge drinking: prevalence, patterns and policy. *Health Educ Res* 1994; 9: 497–505.

11 File S E, Mabbutt P S, Shaffer J. Alcohol consumption and lifestyle in medical students. *J Psycopharmacol* 1994; 8: 22–26.

12 Collier D J, Beales I L P. Drinking among medical students: a questionnaire survey. *Br Med J* 1989; 299: 19–22.

13 Ashton C H, Kamali F. Personality and lifestyles, alcohol and drug consumption in a sample of British medical students. *Med Educ* 1995; 29: 187–92.

14 Gravensten J S, Kong W P, Marks R G: Drug use by anaesthesia personnel and medical students. *Anaesthesiol* 1980; 53: s345.

15 Willis J. The drugs don't work. *BDA Launchpad* 2000: 1: 23–26.

16 The General Dental Council. *Maintaining Standards.* General Dental Council. London, 1997

17 Inter-Departmental Working Group. *Sensible drinking.* Department of Health, London, 1995.

18 Robertson, J A, Plant M A. Alcohol, sex and risk of HIV infection. *Drug and Alcohol Dependence* 1998; 22: 75–78.

19 Bagnal, G. Education as a solution: the need for care, modesty and realism. In Anderton, D. (ed), *Drinking to your Health: The Allegations and the Evidence.* Social Affairs Unit, London, 1990.

20 Home Office Standing Conference on Crime Prevention. *Report of the Working Group on Young People and Alcohol.* Crown Office, London, 1987.

21 Tuck, M. Drinking and disorder: *a study of non-metropolitan violence.* Home Office Research Study 10. HMSO, London, 1980.

22 Kay E, Scarrott D. A survey of dental professionals' health and well-being. *Br Dent J* 1997 183: 340–345.

23 Ritson E B. Teaching medical students about alcohol. *Br Med J* 1990 300: 134–5.

Taking measurements on people 3

The previous chapter introduced some of the main concepts associated with counting people. Here, we provide an introduction to research that involves taking measurements on people (or sometimes objects). Examples of such measurements could be blood pressure, the number of filled teeth or the time taken to recover after oral surgery.

This chapter is not based on a full paper because we concentrate on the interpretation of measurement data rather than study design; measurements can be taken in any type of study. Fundamental to this discussion is the idea of **natural variation**. People are different and any characteristic that we measure will vary from person to person. People have different blood pressures, different numbers of filled teeth and take different times to recover from surgery. This variation must be taken into account when interpreting research. Our discussion of measurements will be based on results from a study that assessed the efficacy of several whitening toothpastes.

Reference: Sharif, N., MacDonald, E., Hughes, J., Newcombe, R.G. and Addy, M. The chemical stain removal properties of 'whitening' toothpaste products: studies *in vitro*. *Br Dent J* 2000;**188**(11):620–624.

The paper was based on taking measurements on acrylic specimens but the same principles apply to studies in which the subjects are people or any other object.

WHAT IS THE AIM OF THE STUDY?

There is a large cosmetics market and people can spend much money on whitening toothpastes, which are usually considerably more expensive than regular ones. Dentists may be asked to recommend one they believe to be effective. Many products are available but being on the market does not necessarily mean that a product is effective. It is important, therefore, to be able to understand and interpret the available information. The aim of this study was to compare the effectiveness of several whitening toothpastes with a regular toothpaste and water alone.

54	65	86	31	39	68	65	58	56	56
29	30	43	44	90	74	78	57	57	53
37	42	46	75	58	59	43	64	69	67

Figure 3.1   Hypothetical data of the effect of a whitening toothpaste (Superdrug Ultracare) on 30 acrylic specimens. Each measurement is the area of stain remaining after 5 minutes (measured in optical density units).

HOW WAS THE STUDY CONDUCTED?

The study by Sharif *et al.* (2000) was based on comparing 28 whitening toothpastes (all available in the shops), seven experimental formulations, one regular toothpaste and water. The authors conducted a series of experiments using acrylic specimens, rather than actual teeth. Each specimen was stained in the same way by being soaked in human saliva for 2 minutes, a 0.2% chlorhexidine mouthrinse for 2 minutes and a tea solution for 60 minutes, repeated until the optical density of the specimens was >2.0.

To test how effective each formulation was at whitening, 3 g of toothpaste gel was mixed in 10 ml of water to form a slurry. An acrylic specimen was then dropped in the mixture (or 15 ml of water, if used alone) in a screw-topped bottle and tumbled for 1 minute, removed and rinsed briefly in water then allowed to dry on the bench. This procedure was repeated four more times, so each specimen was left in the mixture for a total of 5 minutes. Several specimens (three or six) were used for each toothpaste. The main outcome measure was the amount of staining left after 5 minutes, measured using a spectrophotometer – we call the unit of measurement 'optical density unit'.

Understanding natural variation

Figure 3.1 shows hypothetical data from 30 acrylic specimens using the same whitening toothpaste (the data are consistent with the results associated with Superdrug Ultracare, study 1 in the published paper). For the purposes of this discussion the specimens could just as well have been teeth from different people. Each number is the area of staining left after 5 minutes, measured using optical density units. There is a range of values, from 29 to 90 optical density units, even though the same toothpaste was used on all specimens. The effect on the acrylic specimens varies, in the same way that individual teeth from different people would respond differently.

Given these data we now need a way of summarising the efficacy of the toothpaste. We can do this by specifying two measures: one is a value that describes the average (that is, the centre or middle of the data) and the other is a measure of how far the data spread out around the centre. How we describe **average** and **spread** depends on the shape of the data.

We can summarise the data in a table by counting the number of specimens within a particular range of values (Table 3.1). To look at the shape of the data we use the numbers in the table to draw a **histogram** (as shown in Figure 3.2a). This simply shows how many of the specimens take values between certain limits. For example, there are five observations with 40–49 optical density units of stains remaining after 5 minutes.

Table 3.1 Area of stain remaining after 5 minutes for the 30 data values in Figure 3.1. The data are grouped into eight categories (Sharif *et al.*, 2000).

Area of staining (optical density units)	Number of specimens (Frequency)	Percentage
20–29	1	3.3
30–39	4	13.3
40–49	5	16.7
50–59	9	30.0
60–69	6	20.0
70–79	3	10.0
80–89	1	3.3
90–99	1	3.3
Total	30	100.0*

* The actual sum is 99.9%, not 100% due to rounding off of the individual percentages.

The vertical axis could also be converted to a percentage, so 16.7% of observations would be in the range 40–49 optical density units (Figure 3.2b). Whether we draw the histogram based on the number, proportion or percentage of individuals as the vertical axis the shape will be the same. It is usually best to use percentages as the vertical axis because this takes into account the total number of observations in the sample and allows direct comparison of histograms based on different sample sizes.

The histogram in Figure 3.2 looks **symmetric**: there is a fairly even spread on either side of the centre of the data. The measure that best describes the centre of the data

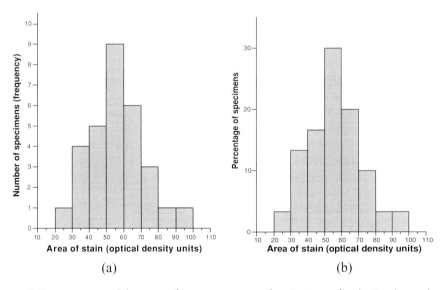

(a) (b)

Figure 3.2 Histogram of the area of stain remaining after 5 minutes for the 30 data values in Table 3.1. The histogram in (a) is based on the number of observations in each staining group (Table 3.2). The histogram in (b) is based on the percentage in each staining group.

Box 3.1

The mean provides a measure of the centre of a distribution of measurements:

$$\text{Mean} = \frac{\text{Sum of all the data values}}{\text{Number of data values}}$$

The standard deviation provides a measure of spread of a distribution about the mean:

$$\text{Standard deviation} = \sqrt{\frac{\text{Sum of (the distance of each data point from the mean)}^2}{\text{Number of data values} - 1}}$$

is the **mean**. To obtain the mean add up the data values and divide by the number of observations. In the example, the sum of the measurements is 1693 and there are 30 observations, so the mean is 56.4 optical density units (1693 ÷ 30), which tells us that the average area of stain remaining is about 56 optical density units.

We have found a mean value for the data, but there are 30 data points each of which is some distance from the mean. How much do the observations spread out about their centre? How much does the level of staining vary between the specimens? The most commonly used measure of spread is the **standard deviation**. This describes the average distance of the data points from the mean value (Box 3.1).

Figure 3.3 illustrates how a standard deviation can be calculated, using five data points. First, we add up the data points and divide by 5 to get the mean value: $(50 + 52 + 57 + 59 + 62) ÷ 5 = 56$. We then calculate how far away each point is from the mean by subtracting the mean from each observation (data value − mean). For example, the data value 52 is −4 optical density units below the mean ($52 − 56 = −4$) and the data value 59 is +3 above the mean ($59 − 56 = +3$).

If we add up all the differences from the mean (−6, −4, +1, +3, +6) the result is 0: the negative numbers cancel out the positive ones because the mean is exactly at the centre of the data. To overcome this we take the square of the differences. The average of these squared differences is $(36 + 16 + 1 + 9 + 36) ÷ 4$, which is 24.5. You might think we divide by the total number of observations, that is, 5, but we actually divide by the number of observations −1 (this is due to a mathematical property associated

Optical density units	50	52	57	59	62
Difference from the mean (56)	−6	−4	+1	+3	+6
Square the ifference	36	16	1	9	36

Sum of the square differences = 98
Divide by (number of observations − 1) = 98/(5 − 1) = 24.5
Take square root to get standard deviation = √24.5 = 4.95

Figure 3.3 Illustration of a standard deviation using five data values.

Table 3.2 Mean and standard deviation of the area of stain remaining after 5 minutes (optical density units) for selected toothpastes and water.

Formulation	Mean	Standard deviation	Number of specimens	Study number
Beverley Hills Natural Whitening	71.0	5.1	6	2
Boots Advanced Whitening	30.1	5.5	6	3
Macleans Whitening	6.4	2.2	6	2
Pearl Drops	63.9	9.1	6	4
Colgate Regular	63.1	6.9	6	2
Water	71.5	11.0	6	4

with calculating a standard deviation in a sample). We then take the square root of the average squared differences to get back to the original scale, giving a standard deviation of 4.95. This tells us that among these data, values differ from the mean by, on average, about 5 optical density units. Looking at the data at Figure 3.3 you can see that this does indeed summarise the average spread.

The standard deviation for the 30 data values in Figure 3.1 is 16 optical density units. This indicates that the values differ from the mean (of 56 optical density units) by, on average, 16 optical density units.

WHAT ARE THE MAIN RESULTS FOR SELECTED TOOTHPASTES AND WATER?

Table 3.2 shows the means and standard deviations for selected whitening toothpastes, taken directly from the published paper by Sharif *et al.* (2000). The effects of the whitening toothpastes are clearly quite variable. Macleans Whitening seems to be most effective because it is associated with the lowest mean area of stain remaining (6.4 optical density units). The standard deviation is 2.2, showing that among the six acrylic samples tested, the values differ from 6.4 by, on average, 2.2 optical density units. Although some of the whitening toothpastes appear to be effective in reducing stain, others seem to be similar to or worse than using a regular toothpaste (Colgate Regular) or even water alone.

We can use the mean values to help us choose between whitening toothpastes. There are formal methods for making such comparisons and these will be considered in Chapter 4.

THE NORMAL DISTRIBUTION

The histogram in Figure 3.2 has a symmetric shape and if a curve is drawn around it, the result is a bell-shaped curve, as shown in Figure 3.4. The curve provides a way of describing a set of measurements (similar to a histogram). This bell-shaped curve is called the **Normal distribution** (or sometimes the Gaussian distribution to avoid

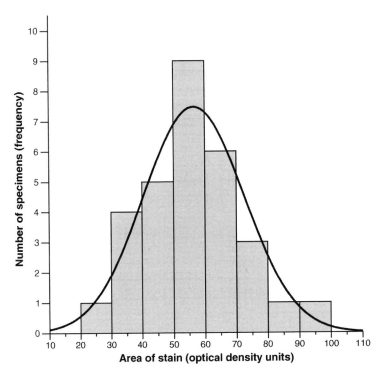

Figure 3.4 Histogram of the area of stain remaining after 5 minutes (optical density units) for the 30 data values in Table 3.1. A smooth bell-shaped curve (Normal distribution) is superimposed.

confusion with standard English usage of the word 'normal'). It is a convenient way of describing the distribution of a measurement. Many measurements in medicine and dentistry have a Normal distribution.

The Normal distribution has some useful mathematical properties. In particular, if we know the mean and the standard deviation of the data there is a formula which enables us to draw the bell-shaped curve. If the curve was derived from a histogram, it would need to be based on several hundred observations to produce a smooth histogram. Because the Normal distribution curve can be derived from just the mean and standard deviation, when we only have a few observations we can still get a picture of the data.

Using the mean and standard deviation obtained from the 30 (hypothetical) data values in Figure 3.1 (mean 56 and standard deviation 16 optical density units), the resulting Normal curve is shown in Figure 3.5. The horizontal axis (x-axis) is the measurement of interest; here it is the area of stain remaining after 5 minutes and the vertical axis (y-axis) comes from the formula for the Normal distribution.[1] The Normal curve is a useful way of graphically displaying the average level and spread at the same time.

---

[1] The formula for the Normal distribution is complicated for those who are unfamiliar with it, but we do not need to deal with it here.

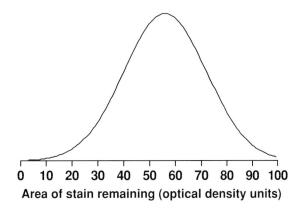

Area of stain remaining (optical density units)

Figure 3.5 Normal distribution curve for Superdrug Ultracare.

The implications of conducting a study based on a sample of people

In Chapter 2, the concepts of **population** and **sample** were introduced. We wanted to know information about a large population of people, that is all dental undergraduates in the UK in 1998, but the study was based on only a sample. We used the observed data from the sample to estimate parameters (in this case prevalence) in the population. The same principle applies here. The main parameter of interest is the mean area of stain remaining after five minutes and this is measured in samples of size six. The question is, therefore, what is the **true** mean value? This would be the mean obtained from a study based on *every* acrylic specimen ever. Such a study is clearly impossible to do, but we can use our sample mean to estimate the true mean and use **confidence intervals** to tell us how good our estimate is likely to be, given the sample size.

In standard English usage the word population refers to the inhabitants of a geographical area. In research, **population** refers to the set of all people (or specimens) that we are interested in studying. When we take a **sample** from the **population** we want to use it to make inferences not just about the individuals in the sample, but about the whole of the population of interest. In dentistry and medicine we often study people who have a particular disease and we want to make statements not just about the people in our sample, but about everyone who has the disease or may get it in the future. For example when we research a new drug to alleviate pain in children having dental treatment, we test it on a sample of children, but we want to know how the drug will perform on all children, now and in the future. We can never study the population of all children. When we move from considering a sample to considering the population from which it comes, there is always some uncertainty in what we can infer about the population from the sample. We have methods of describing this uncertainty: one of the most powerful of these is the **confidence interval**.

As we saw with proportions (see Figure 2.1 in Chapter 2), we expect the proportion of people with a particular characteristic to vary from study to study (that is, from sample to sample). Furthermore, the smaller the sample size from which we calculate the proportion the more uncertain we will be that our observed estimate is close to the true value (see Figure 2.2 in Chapter 2). These principles are the same for any statistic we are interested in, including the mean value. Whatever we measure will have a different value if we take another sample, and the more people we measure the more certain we are that our sample measurement reflects the true population value.

Figure 3.6 shows the mean area of stain remaining and its confidence interval for 20 hypothetical studies of Superdrug Ultracare. Study 1 comes from the data in Figure 3.1 (mean value of 56, standard deviation of 16 and sample size of 30 observations). Each study is based on the same number of acrylic samples but each has a different

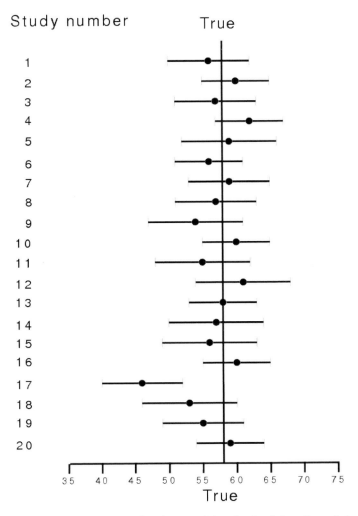

Mean area of stain remaining (optical density units)

Figure 3.6 The mean and 95% confidence interval for 20 hypothetical studies of the whitening toothpaste Superdrug Ultracare (the result for study 1 comes from the data in Figure 3.1). The true mean is assumed to be 58 optical density units.

Box 3.2

For the $n = 30$ data values in Figure 3.1
Mean area of stain remaining $= \bar{x} = 56$ optical density units
Standard deviation of the data $= s = 16$ optical density units

$$\text{Standard error of the mean (SE)} = \frac{s}{\sqrt{n}} = \frac{16}{\sqrt{30}} = 2.9 \text{ optical density units}$$

(The mean and standard deviation for a sample are often notated by $\bar{x}$ and s, respectively)

mean. Each study and its 95% confidence interval aims to estimate the true mean value which, for the purposes of this discussion, we assume is known to be 58 optical density units. Some studies have a mean value that is above 58 and others below, but all the confidence intervals include the true mean except study 17. This is expected. A 95% confidence interval indicates that the range will contain the true mean about 95% of the time but it will miss the true mean 5% of the time (that is 1 in 20 studies).

The variability of a statistic (be it a proportion or mean) can be quantified by the **standard error**. It is a measure of the uncertainty associated with trying to estimate the **true** value when we only have a sample of specimens (or people) in our study. So the standard error of the mean measures how much the mean is likely to vary from sample to sample. An important application of the standard error is that we can use it to calculate a confidence interval.

It is easy to calculate the standard error for a mean. It is found by taking the standard deviation for the sample and dividing it by the square root of the number of observations in the sample. People sometimes get confused between standard deviation and standard error. Standard deviation tells us how much the data in our sample is spread out about the mean. Standard error is related not to the spread of the data but to the accuracy with which we have been able to calculate our summary statistic (here, the mean value) (Box 3.2).

For the data in Figure 3.1, the centre of the data is at 56 optical density units and the data spreads either side of it by, on average, 16 optical density units. The standard error is 2.9, so if we had several studies, each based on 30 acrylic specimens, the means from these would have a spread of about 2.9 about the true mean. We use the standard error of the mean to calculate the 95% confidence interval for the mean (Box 3.3).

Box 3.3

Calculating the confidence interval (CI) for a mean

Lower limit of CI = observed mean − (1.96 × standard error)
Upper limit of CI = observed mean + (1.96 × standard error)

1.96 is used when there are about 30 or more observations; for smaller samples the multiplier used is slightly larger and will depend on the sample size

Table 3.3 Mean and 95% confidence interval of the area of stain remaining after 5 minutes (optical density units) for selected toothpastes and water (Sharif *et al.*, 2000).

Formulation	Mean	95% confidence interval
Beverley Hills Natural Whitening	71.0	65.6 to 76.3
Boots Advanced Whitening	30.1	24.3 to 35.9
Macleans Whitening	6.4	4.1 to 8.7
Pearl Drops	63.9	54.3 to 73.4
Colgate Regular	63.1	55.9 to 70.3
Water	71.5	60.0 to 83.0

Using the results from our 30 data values in Figure 3.1, where the observed mean is 56 and standard error is 2.9, the 95% confidence interval is 50 to 62. We use this information to say that our best estimate for the **true** mean for the toothpaste Superdrug Ultracare is 56 optical density units but whatever the true mean is we are 95% sure that it is somewhere between 50 and 62.

Table 3.3 shows the mean and 95% confidence intervals for the toothpastes specified in Table 3.2. For example, the true mean for Pearl Drops is likely to lie in the range 54.3–73.4, while the true mean for water is likely to lie in the range 60.0–83.0. These two intervals overlap greatly, which implies that Pearl Drops and water could have the same effect on stain removal. Formal ways of comparing two toothpastes are discussed in Chapter 4.

INTERPRETING THE RESULTS FROM NON-SYMMETRIC DATA

The principles presented above are associated with data that is symmetric; a histogram of such data spreads evenly about its centre. Measurements whose distribution is not symmetric cannot be represented by a Normal distribution. An example of this is biteforce. Figure 3.7 shows a histogram based on the biteforce measurement (measured in newtons, N) of 500 women. The shape is not symmetric, but rather it is **skewed** to the left (other measurements may be skewed to the right). In these situations the mean value will not give us a good estimate of the centre of the data.

The **median** is the value that has half the data points below it and half above. In Figure 3.7 the median is the value that has 250 data points below it and 250 above. This is 400 N. The mean value is 480 N, larger than the median because it is influenced by the relatively few women who have very high values. When data are not symmetric, the centre is best described by the median.

Similarly, the spread of skewed data is not best represented by the standard deviation. To illustrate this consider the eight data values:

11,   12,   13,   14,   15,   16,   17,   100

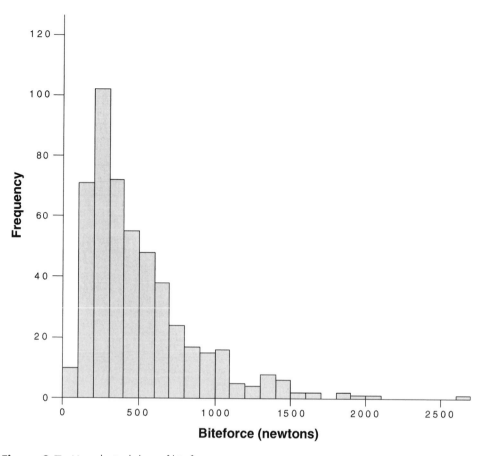

Figure 3.7 Hypothetical data of biteforce measurements in 500 women.

The standard deviation is 30, which clearly does not represent the average spread between most of the data values which are centred around 14. Like the mean, the standard deviation will be influenced by very large (or small) values. When the data are not symmetric, the spread is best represented by the **interquartile range**. This is the distance between the 25th and 75th centile. The 50th centile is the median.

The 25th centile is the value below which 25% of the data lie and the 75th centile is the value below which 75% of the data lie (therefore 25% of the data lie above). For the example of the eight data values, 25% of the data is two data values (25% × 8), so the 25th centile is between the second and third values, that is, about 12.5. The 75th centile has two data points above and so is between the sixth and seventh values; about 16.5. Therefore the interquartile range is from 12.5 to 16.5 which is 4 (Figure 3.8). Box 3.4 compares the different measures of average and spread for this set of eight data values.

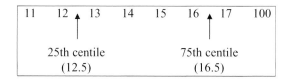

Figure 3.8 Eight hypothetical data values and the estimation of the 25th and 75th centiles.

Box 3.4

Mean	24.8	The median is closer to the
Median	14.5	centre of the data than the mean
Standard Deviation	30	The inter-quartile range gives a better
Inter-quartile range	4	idea of spread than the standard deviation

In the example of 500 women, the 25th centile is the biteforce measurement below which there are 125 values (25% of 500); this is 243 N. The 75th centile is 588 N (that is, there are 125 values above it). So half of the women have biteforce measurements between 243 N and 588 N. The interquartile range is therefore 345 N (588 − 243).

Because the data is skewed the median and interquartile range give a better description of the data than the mean and standard deviation.

Key points

- Measurements on people involve natural variation.
- Centre and spread are both needed to describe measurements on a group of people.
  - ○ Mean and standard deviation are used if the data are symmetrical (Normally distributed).
  - ○ Median and interquartile range are used if the data are skewed (not Normally distributed).
- A confidence interval for a mean provides a range within which the true (population) mean is likely to lie.

Exercise

(1) The 40 hypothetical observations in the box below show the amount of stain remaining (in optical density units) associated with a whitening toothpaste in 40 acrylic samples. Calculate the mean, median and interquartile range.

28	19	43	26	28	41	30	31	29	29
26	22	33	31	23	37	30	27	34	34
27	35	30	31	27	28	27	25	29	36
27	23	41	33	31	29	33	27	30	30

(2) From the data above, the standard deviation is 5.05 optical density units. What does this tell us?

(3) Do you think the distribution is symmetric or skewed? Depending on your answer, what are the most appropriate measures of average and spread to describe these data?

(4) Calculate the standard error of the mean.

(5) What is the 95% confidence interval for the true mean for this particular whitening toothpaste? Interpret the results.

(6) If we had only 15 observations instead of 40, what would be the effect on the 95% confidence intrval?

Answers on pp. 209–210

Comparing groups of people and examining associations

The previous two chapters were based on describing the characteristics of a group of people (or objects) either by counting them or measuring something on them. This was done by estimating a proportion (percentage) or a mean for a *single* group of people.

Investigating a new treatment for or cause of oral disease will involve *comparing* characteristics between two or more groups. We cannot tell if a new treatment for periodontitis is effective unless we make some comparison with a group of people who did not have the new treatment. Similarly, to determine whether smoking is a cause of oral cancer we can only tell that the risk in smokers is raised if we compare it with the risk in non-smokers.

In Chapter 2 we introduced the concepts of relative risk and absolute risk difference, both of which involve comparing two percentages. In this chapter we expand on this and introduce the comparison of two means. The first two sections of this chapter are based on results that have already been presented in Chapters 2 and 3. In the last section we introduce a method of investigating associations. This chapter covers some of the fundamental concepts that will be used in later chapters.

COMPARING TWO PERCENTAGES (OR PROPORTIONS)

In the paper discussed in Chapter 2, the authors describe the prevalence of students who binge drink (*Table 1* of the paper by Underwood and Fox; see p. 27). Looking at the results for female students only, we can create a table in which binge drinking can be compared between the different years of study (Table 4.1). For female students, the risk of being a binge drinker in Years 1–3 is 69% and the risk of being a binge drinker in Years 4–5 is 39%. This means the relative risk of binge drinking in Years 1–3 compared with Years 4–5 is 69/39 = 1.8. That is, female students in Years 1–3 are 1.8 times (or almost twice) as likely to binge drink as those in Years 4–5.

A relative risk compares the risk in one group with that of another, so when interpreting a relative risk you need to be clear what the comparison group is. For example, it is not meaningful to say, 'Female students in Years 1–3 are twice as likely to binge drink'. You need further information: 'Female students in Years 1–3 are twice

Table 4.1 Binge drinking among 100 female students according to year of study (Underwood and Fox, 2000).

	Female students Number (%)	
Binge drinking	**Years 1–3**	**Years 4–5**
Yes	44 (69)	14 (39)*
No	20 (31)	22 (61)
	64 (100)	36 (100)

* Reported as 40.0% in *Table 1*.

as likely to binge drink *compared to those in Years 4–5'*. The group that we are comparing against is called the **reference group**, and we can choose which group we want as the reference. In the example above, the reference group is Years 4–5. What would happen if we had taken Years 1–3 as the reference group? The relative risk would be $39/69 = 0.56$. This is interpreted as 'Female students in Years 4–5 are *about half* as likely to binge drink as those in Years 1–3'.

What would the relative risk be if binge drinking were unrelated to year of study? In this case the percentage of female students would be the same in both groups. If two risks are exactly the same, dividing one by the other will produce a relative risk of one. We call this value the **no effect value** for the relative risk.

Another way of comparing binge drinking between the different years of study is to look at the **absolute risk difference**, found by subtracting the two percentages. This would be $69\% - 39\% = 30\%$, that is, 30% more of the female students in Years 1–3 binge drink than those in Years 4–5. So, if there were 100 female students in Years 1–3 and 100 in Years 4–5, there would be an *extra* 30 who binge drink in Years 1–3. Again, the reference group consists of Years 4–5. We could have chosen Years 1–3 as the reference group. This would give us an absolute risk difference of $39\% - 69\% = -30\%$. The minus sign tells us that there are 30% fewer females in Years 4–5 who binge drink than those in Years 1–3. What would the **no effect value** be for the absolute risk difference? If the percentage of binge drinkers was the same in each study year, because we are subtracting one risk from another for the risk difference the **no effect value** would be 0.

When interpreting relative risks or risk differences we need to look carefully at the comparison that is being made and be sure which group is taken as the reference. Whichever way we do it the magnitude of the difference stays the same, it is just in a different direction, in that twice as risky is the inverse of half as risky, and 30% more at risk is the converse of 30% less at risk. In Table 4.2 we summarise the comparisons between binge drinking in different years among female students.

The relative risk (or risk difference) indicates the magnitude of the effect, but not whether the effect is beneficial or harmful; this depends on the nature of the outcome measure used. If the outcome is positive, such as the percentage of people who are alive or the percentage of children who are caries-free, a relative risk that is greater

Table 4.2 Specifying the reference group and the effect on relative risk and risk difference (Underwood and Fox, 2000).

Comparison	Reference group	Relative risk (RR) or Absolute risk difference (ARD)
Years 1–3 are twice as likely to drink as Years 4–5	Years 4–5	RR = 1.8 (or 1/0.56)
Years 4–5 are half as likely to drink as Years 1–3	Years 1–3	RR = 0.56 (or 1/1.8)
30% more drink in Years 1–3 than Years 4–5	Years 4–5	ARD = 30%
30% fewer drink in Years 4–5 than Years 1–3	Years 1–3	ARD = −30%

than one indicates benefit. If the outcome is negative, such as the percentage of people who are dead or the percentage of people who experience pain after oral surgery, a relative risk greater than one indicates harm. Box 4.1 illustrates this.

The implications of conducting a study based on a sample of people

In Chapter 2, a 95% confidence interval was calculated for a single observed proportion, giving us a measure of the precision with which we were able to estimate the **true proportion**. We are often interested in comparing proportions in different groups, where the statistic of most interest to us summarises the *comparison* between the groups, telling us how much they differ. We found that the risk of binge drinking among female students is 69% in Years 1–3 and 39% in Years 4–5, giving us a risk difference of 30%. If we could obtain data on the drinking habits of all female dental students in the UK in 1998 we would get the **true** risk difference.

Box 4.1

Outcome measure: percentage of patients who recover from gingivitis after 1 month

Antibiotic A	Antibiotic B	Relative risk
90%	70%	1.3 (90/70)
		Antibiotic A is better than antibiotic B

Outcome measure: percentage of patients who experience pain after dental surgery

Treatment C	Treatment D	Relative risk
40%	20%	2.0 (40/20)
		Treatment C is worse than treatment D

The risk difference observed in our sample is only an estimate of the true risk difference. What would happen if we took another sample – how large would the observed risk difference be? It is unlikely to be exactly the same as that in our current sample, so we need to have some idea about how much risk differences are likely to vary between samples. The **standard error** of the risk difference tells us how much it is likely to vary from sample to sample and gives us a measure of the uncertainty associated with the risk difference when we are trying to estimate its true value. The standard error for the risk difference in the example is about 10%. How it is calculated is not of interest here, only its interpretation and use. (Details can be found in books on epidemiology and medical statistics in Further Reading). If we took several other samples of female students of the same size the risk differences are likely to vary by, on average, 10%. The standard error allows us to construct a confidence interval (Box 4.2). For the risk difference of 30%, found in our sample, the 95% confidence interval is 10% to 50%. So our best estimate of the true difference in binge drinking between the different years of study is 30%. The confidence interval gives us a range within which we are fairly sure the true difference will lie. In this case the confidence interval is quite wide: the true difference could be as low as 10% or as high as 50%, so there is a lot of uncertainty in our estimate. The risk difference can only take values from -100% to $+100\%$.

Because every statistic that we measure will have a standard error, indicating how much it varies from sample to sample, we can always calculate a confidence interval for a statistic.

Box 4.2

The calculation for a 95% confidence interval (CI) for an absolute risk difference (ARD) is straightforward:

Lower limit of CI = observed ARD − (1.96 × standard error of ARD)

Upper limit of CI = observed ARD + (1.96 × standard error of ARD)

The calculation for a 95% confidence interval for a relative risk (RR) is based on first taking the logarithm of the relative risk, then taking the antilog of the result:

Lower limit of CI = antilog [log observed RR − (1.96 × standard error of log RR)]

Upper limit of CI = antilog [log observed RR + (1.96 × standard error of log RR)]

> **Box 4.3**
>
> Binge drinking in females in Years 1–3 compared with Years 4–5
>
> Absolute risk difference = 30%   95% confidence interval is 10% to 50%
>
> Relative risk = 1.8   95% confidence interval is 1.1 to 2.8

The other method we used to compare binge drinking in the two groups was the relative risk (estimated to be 1.8); female students in Years 1–3 are 1.8 times as likely to be binge drinkers than those in Years 4–5. The relative risk, like the risk difference, will vary from sample to sample and we can find its standard error and use this to construct a confidence interval (Box 4.2). The 95% confidence interval for the true relative risk is 1.1 to 2.8. We are never going to know exactly what the true relative risk is, but there is a 95% chance that it lies somewhere between 1.1 and 2.8 (Box 4.3). The possible range of relative risk values is infinite, unlike that for the risk difference.

Is the observed effect a chance finding?

In the example above, there is a 30% difference in the prevalence of binge drinking between Years 1–3 and Years 4–5 among female students. This looks like quite a large difference, but can we be sure that it reflects a *real* difference in the underlying population? If our study were based on *every* UK female dental undergraduate would we see a difference as large as 30% between the prevalences, or could there, in fact, be no difference at all? Could the observed result of 30% be just a chance finding in this particular study? To help determine this we use a **statistical test**, which produces a **p-value**. When comparing two or more proportions or percentages a test called a chi-squared (χ^2) test is often used to calculate a p-value. Details of this test and how to calculate p-values are not discussed in this book because the aim here is to concentrate on interpretation. (See books on epidemiology and medical statistics in Further Reading.) The chi-squared test compares the difference between the two prevalences, taking into account the sample size on which each prevalence is based.

The p-value associated with a difference of 30% (69% versus 39%), when each percentage is based on 64 and 36 students, respectively, is 0.003. We interpret this as follows. If the study had been based on every female dental student in the UK in 1998 and there was no difference at all between the prevalence of binge drinking between the years of study, the **true difference** would be 0 (**no effect value** is 0). Even when the true difference is 0, if there were several studies based on different samples of people we could occasionally see a difference of 30% or more just due to chance. The p-value of 0.003 tells us that a difference this large would only occur in 3 in 1000 studies of the same size just by chance alone, if there were no real difference. This means that our observed result (30% difference) is unlikely to arise by chance. The difference we have observed between the years of study is likely to reflect a real effect.

Box 4.4

Difference between two proportions (absolute risk difference)	If p-value ≤0.05 observed risk difference is statistically significant	The true difference is unlikely to be 0; there is likely to be a real effect
No effect value = 0	If p-value >0.05 observed risk difference is not statistically significant	We do not have enough evidence to say that there is an effect
Ratio of two proportions (relative risk)	If p-value ≤0.05 observed relative risk is statistically significant	The true relative risk is unlikely to be 1; there is likely to be a real effect
No effect value = 1	If p-value >0.05 observed relative risk is not statistically significant	We do not have enough evidence to say that there is an effect

The p-value is always in the range 0 to 1. By convention, if the p-value is ≤0.05 we say that the observed result is **statistically significant** and is unlikely to have arisen just by chance. If the p-value is >0.05 we say the result is **not statistically significant** and there is no evidence for a true difference. Finding a result that is not statistically significant is *not* the same as concluding that there is no effect, it only indicates that we do not have enough evidence to say that there is an effect (Box 4.4).

When making comparisons there is always a relationship between confidence intervals and p-values (Box 4.5). A confidence interval that does not contain the no effect value will mean that the result is statistically significant (the p-value is ≤0.05). If the confidence interval contains the no effect value then the p-value will be >0.05, and the result will not be statistically significant. In the past, researchers tended to report only the p-value and not confidence intervals. However, both are useful. The p-value tells us how likely it is that our result arose by chance alone and the confidence interval provides a range of the possible size of the true effect.

Alternative interpretation of relative risk

When the relative risk is much larger than one, the idea of twice or ten times as likely is easy to understand and explain. However, when the relative risk is less than two it can be more difficult to interpret; 1.15 times the risk may not be intuitively meaningful. Relative risk is therefore sometimes expressed as a percentage change in risk because this is easier to explain. This is often referred to as the **relative risk reduction** if the relative risk is less than one or **excess relative risk** (sometimes just **excess risk**) if it is above one.

The percentage change in risk is the difference between two risks expressed as a percentage of the risk in the reference group. For example, if the risk was 20% in

Box 4.5

Relative risk
No effect value = 1

If the 95% confidence interval contains 1 this implies p >0.05	If p >0.05 this implies the confidence interval contains 1
If the 95% confidence interval does not contain 1 this implies p ≤0.05	If p ≤0.05 this implies the confidence interval does not contain 1

Risk difference
No effect value = 0

If the 95% confidence interval contains 0 this implies p >0.05	If p >0.05 this implies the confidence interval contains 0
If the 95% confidence interval does not contain 0 this implies p ≤0.05	If p ≤0.05 this implies the confidence interval does not contain 0

group A and 50% in group B, and group B is taken as the reference, the absolute risk difference is $20\% - 50\%$ which is -30%. The negative sign simply tells us that the risk in group A is lower than in group B. The percentage change in risk, or **risk reduction**, would be 60% calculated as $(-30/50) \times 100$. This can also be calculated directly from the relative risk (Box 4.6).

The relative risk of group A compared with group B is 0.4, so the risk reduction is $(0.4 - 1) \times 100 = -60\%$. The risk in group A is reduced by 60% compared with the risk in group B (Box 4.6). Similarly, a relative risk of 1.35 can be interpreted as an **excess risk** of 35%; the risk in group A is increased by 35% compared with the risk in group B.

When the relative risk is greater than 2 the equivalent percentage change looks cumbersome. For example, the relative risk of getting lung cancer in cigarette smokers

Box 4.6

Risk in group A = R_A
Risk in group B = R_B

$$\text{Percentage change in risk} = [(R_A - R_B)/R_B] \times 100$$
$$= [R_A/R_B - R_B/R_B] \times 100$$
$$= [R_A/R_B - 1] \times 100$$
$$= (\text{Relative risk} - 1) \times 100$$

Risk in group A = 20%
Risk in group B = 50%

$$\text{Percentage change in risk} = [(20 - 50)/50] \times 100$$
$$= -60\%$$
$$(\text{Relative risk} - 1) \times 100 = (0.4 - 1) \times 100$$
$$= -60\%$$

is about 20. This would be equivalent to a 1900% increase in risk: ($[20 − 1] \times 100$). When the relative risk is large, it is therefore not necessary to convert to a percentage change. It is sufficient to say twice as likely (relative risk of 2) or 20 times as likely (relative risk of 20).

COMPARING TWO MEANS

In Chapter 3 we discussed the efficacy of individual whitening toothpastes. Now we wish to make comparisons between them. Table 4.3 shows the results for several toothpastes and water. The following questions could be asked:

- Is Boots Advanced Whitening better than Beverley Hills Natural Whitening?
- Is Macleans Whitening better than water?
- Is Pearl Drops similar to water?
- Is Pearl Drops similar to a regular toothpaste, Colgate Regular?

The discussion presented below is based only on the results presented in this one paper and refers only to the limited evidence provided by this particular experiment on staining acrylic samples, where each experiment only included a small number of samples. The results should not be taken as definitive evidence of the effectiveness of any of the products described.

First, to get a picture of the effects of the toothpastes we can use the means and standard deviations to draw the Normal distribution curves. Figure 4.1 shows the distributions of Beverley Hills Natural Whitening and Boots Advanced Whitening together and the distribution of Pearl Drops and Colgate Regular. We can judge by eye what each comparison tells us. Figure 4.1a clearly shows that in this study Boots Advanced Whitening is better than Beverley Hills Natural Whitening, the curves hardly overlap. Figure 4.1b shows that Pearl Drops looks very similar to Colgate Regular as the curves lie almost on top of one another. However, there needs to be an objective criterion for helping us to make decisions about effectiveness; **statistical tests** provide us with this.

Table 4.3 Mean and standard deviation of the area of stain remaining after 5 minutes (optical density units) (Sharif *et al.*, 2000).

Formulation	Mean	Standard deviation	Number of samples
Beverley Hills Natural Whitening	71.0	5.1	6
Boots Advanced Whitening	30.1	5.5	6
Macleans Whitening	6.4	2.2	6
Pearl Drops	63.9	9.1	6
Colgate Regular	63.1	6.9	6
Water	71.5	11.0	6

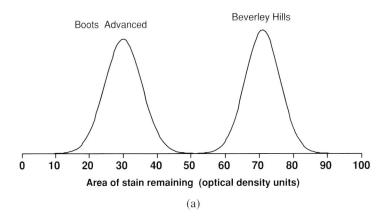

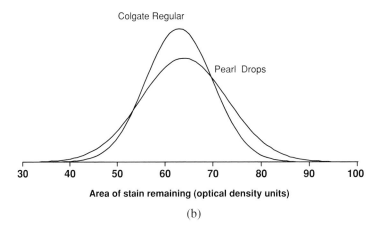

Figure 4.1   The Normal distribution curves for four whitening toothpastes: Boots Advanced versus Beverley Hills (a) and Colgate Regular versus Pearl Drops (b).

Is the observed effect a chance finding?

Earlier in this chapter we used a statistical test to compare two percentages. Other tests exist to compare two means or two medians if the data do not have a Normal distribution. (See books on epidemiology and medical statistics in Further Reading.) For our purposes, the p-value, which the test produces, is of importance because this is what we interpret. To answer the question of whether Boots Advanced Whitening is better than Beverley Hills Natural Whitening, we look at the difference between the mean area of stain remaining after 5 minutes. The mean values were 30.1 and 71.0 optical density units respectively; a difference of about 41 units. We then perform a statistical test (called a *t*-test) on the difference. The *t*-test compares the difference between the two means, taking into account both the sample size on which each mean is based and the standard deviation in each group. The test gives a p-value of <0.001, but what does this tell us?

Box 4.7

	If p-value ≤0.05 observed difference in means is statistically significant	The true difference in means is unlikely to be 0; there is likely to be a real effect
Difference between two means		
No effect value = 0	If p-value >0.05 observed difference in means is not statistically significant	We do not have enough evidence to say that there is an effect

If the two toothpastes really have exactly the same effect on staining the **true difference** between the means would be 0 (**no effect value** is 0). Even when the true difference is 0, if we had several different studies then we could occasionally see a difference of 41 optical density units or more just due to chance. The p-value tells us that a difference this large would occur in less than 1 in 1000 studies of the same size just by chance alone, if the true difference were 0. This means that the observed result (a difference of 41 optical density units) is unlikely to arise by chance, so the difference observed between the two toothpastes is likely to reflect a real effect. We can say that the study gives us evidence that Boots Advanced Whitening really does remove more stain than Beverley Hills Whitening. The smaller the p-value the more certain we become that there is a real effect (Box 4.7), and p-values that are very small, for example <0.001, are often described as *highly statistically significant*.

The implications of conducting a study based on a sample of people

In Chapter 3 we calculated confidence intervals for the individual means, because we know they will vary from sample to sample. The statistic we are really interested in here is the **difference in two means** for different toothpastes because this tells us by how much, on average, one toothpaste is better than another. We found that the difference in means between Boots Advanced Whitening and Beverley Hills Whitening was 41 optical density units. If we took another sample, this would give us another estimate of the difference in means. So we express the uncertainty in our estimate in a confidence interval. The 95% confidence interval for the **true difference** is 34 to 48 optical density units. We interpret this result by saying that given the present study, our best estimate of the true difference is 41 optical density units and we are 95% sure that the true difference lies somewhere between 34 and 48 optical density units.

If the two means are identical, indicating the two toothpastes have the same effect, the difference between them will be 0 (the **no effect value**). We therefore see whether the confidence interval contains 0 or not. If it does this implies that the two toothpastes might be equally effective. Our confidence interval of 34 to 48 optical density units does not contain 0, so we think it unlikely that the toothpastes have the same effect.

Box 4.8

Differences in means or medians

No effect value = 0

If the 95% confidence interval contains 0 this implies p >0.05	If p >0.05 this implies the confidence interval contains 0
If the 95% confidence interval does not contain 0 this implies p ≤0.05	If p ≤0.05 this implies the confidence interval does not contain 0

This is consistent with the p-value being <0.05, which also tells us that the true means are unlikely to be the same. There is always a relationship between confidence intervals and p-values (Box 4.8).

Table 4.4 shows the 95% confidence intervals and p-values for the difference associated with selected comparisons from Table 4.3. The difference between the mean measurements, the 95% confidence interval and the p-value can all be used to interpret the results. Below are conclusions that may be drawn about the comparisons in Table 4.4:

- Boots Advanced is better at whitening than Beverley Hills. There is a large difference between the means (about 41 optical density units), which is highly statistically

Table 4.4 Comparison of selected whitening toothpastes (Sharif *et al.*, 2000).

Comparison of toothpastes (mean area of stain remaining after 5 minutes, optical density units) A vs B	Difference between the means) (mean A − mean B)	95% CI for the difference	p-value
Beverley Hills (71.0) vs Boots Advanced (30.1)	40.9	34.1 to 47.8	<0.001
Pearl Drops (63.9) vs Colgate Regular (63.1)	0.8	−9.6 to 11.2	0.86
Beverley Hills (71.0) vs Colgate Regular (63.1)	7.9	0.1 to 15.7	0.048
Pearl Drops (63.9) vs Water (71.5)	−7.6	−20.6 to 5.4	0.22

The measure of effectiveness is the area of stain remaining. When we look at the difference between the means:

- a *positive* value implies the first toothpaste is *worse* than the second (mean A > mean B)
- a *negative* value implies the first toothpaste is *better* than the second (mean A < mean B)

significant, that is, the difference is unlikely to be due to chance. The true difference is expected to lie somewhere between 34 and 48 optical density units, in favour of Boots Advanced. The lower limit of the 95% confidence interval is far from 0, so the smallest advantage achievable using Boots Advanced is expected to be 34 optical density units.

- There is no evidence that Pearl Drops is better or worse than Colgate Regular. The difference between the means is small, 0.8 optical density units, and close to 0, and the 95% confidence interval covers a range that includes 0. The p-value of 0.86 indicates that if there were no underlying difference, we could see a difference as large as 0.8 (or more) in 86 out of 100 similar studies just by chance alone. This result is therefore not statistically significant; the difference of 0.8 could easily have arisen by natural variation between samples.

- Colgate Regular is, on average, about 8 optical density units better than Beverley Hills. The result is just statistically significant (p-value is 0.048). The 95% confidence interval indicates that the true difference could be as low as 0.1 optical density units and as high as 15.7. However, although these results indicate that there is a real difference between these toothpastes, the effect may not be sufficiently large to recommend one over the other. The result, while statistically significant, may not be considered **clinically important**.

- There is insufficient evidence to conclude that Pearl Drops is better than water. The difference is −7.6 optical density units, with a p-value of 0.22. Even though the result is not statistically significant, the confidence interval may provide further information on effectiveness. The confidence interval is −20.6 to +5.4, and although it includes 0, most of the range is negative, that is, in favour of Pearl Drops, by up to −20.6. If the true difference were as much as 20 optical density units in favour of Pearl Drops, this could be clinically important. Because this study was small, the researchers could decide to conduct a larger one to look at this effect more closely. Confidence intervals can show an important effect which could be missed if conclusions were based only on the p-value.

For many results seen in the literature, the 95% confidence interval and p-values will provide the information on which we base formal comparisons. Confidence intervals are useful because they provide a range of the possible true effect sizes based on the sample of data, whereas p-values indicate the likelihood that differences as large as the ones we see in our sample may have arisen just by chance, if there were no real underlying difference.

EXAMINING ASSOCIATIONS

The methods described in the previous section can be used to compare a single measurement between two groups of people. In this section we discuss how to examine associations between two measurements taken on the same person or object. First we use a simple example to illustrate the method and then look at how this has been

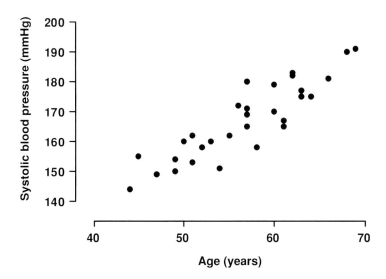

Figure 4.2   Scatter plot of age and systolic blood pressure in 30 men in the UK.

applied in dentistry using a paper on water fluoridation, poverty and tooth decay. The example we use to illustrate the method is blood pressure and age measured on 30 men in England. There are two questions we wish to answer:

• If we know a man's age can this help us predict his blood pressure?
• How strong is the relationship between blood pressure and age?

The techniques that allow us to answer these questions are, respectively, **linear regression** and **correlation**.

Linear regression

Figure 4.2 is a **scatter plot** of blood pressure measurement and age for 30 men aged 40–70 years in England. If there was no association between blood pressure and age the observations would tend to lie horizontally, showing neither an increase nor a decrease with age. However, we can see that there is a tendency for blood pressure to increase with increasing age.

How much, on average, does blood pressure increase for each year of age? We can answer this question by fitting a straight line through the data. There are mathematical techniques for finding the equation of the straight line that best represents the data. The line that, on average, is closest to all the points is called the **linear regression** line. The regression line for blood pressure and age is shown in Figure 4.3.

To interpret this we need to understand the equation for a straight line. The linear regression equation always has the form shown in Box 4.9. In our example the line in

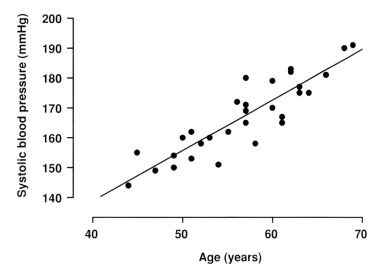

Figure 4.3 Scatter plot of age and systolic blood pressure in 30 men in the UK, with a regression line fitted through the data points.

Figure 4.3 has the following form:

$$\text{Systolic blood pressure} = 71 + (1.7 \times \text{age})$$

Using the equation we can work out what the average level of blood pressure is at any age.

- At age 50 years: average blood pressure $= 71 + (1.7 \times 50) = 156\,\text{mmHg}$
- At age 60 years: average blood pressure $= 71 + (1.7 \times 60) = 173\,\text{mmHg}$

The slope of the line, 1.7, in the regression line above is illustrated in Figure 4.4. It is represented by J/I. I is an increase in age of 10 years, from age 50 to 60. J is an

---

Box 4.9

$$y = a + bx$$

- x is the measurement on the horizontal axis (x-axis), here $x =$ age
- y is the measurement on the vertical axis (y-axis), here $y =$ blood pressure
- b is the slope of the line and is called the regression coefficient. It quantifies the rate of change in y for a change in x of 1 unit
- a is the intercept term. It is the value of the y measurement when $x = 0$

---

increase in blood pressure of 17 mmHg, from 156 to 173. So the slope of the line is $1.7 = 17/10$. The estimate of slope of 1.7 means that for every increase in age of one

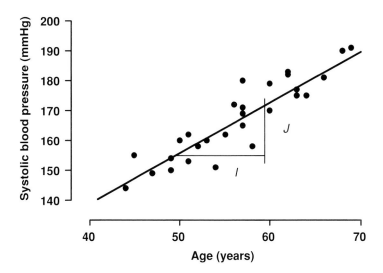

Figure 4.4   Scatter plot of age and systolic blood pressure in 30 men in the UK, with a regression line fitted through the data points. The width *I* represents a difference of 10 years of age and this is associated with an increase of blood pressure of 17 mmHg (the height *J*). The slope of the regression line is *J* ÷ *I*.

year, blood pressure is expected to increase by 1.7 mmHg. This might seem a small change but we can use it to estimate the increase in blood pressure for an increase of say 5 or 10 years. For a 5-year age difference blood pressure increases by 8.5 mmHg (1.7 × 5), and for a 10-year difference, it increases by 17 mmHg (1.7 × 10).

The regression line comes from a *sample* of observations, but we want to be able to make inferences about the association between age and blood pressure in the whole *population* of interest; for our example, this would be *all* men in England aged 40–70 years. As with any other statistic that we have covered so far (percentage, relative risk, mean and difference between two means) the slope will have an associated **standard error**; we can use this to estimate a 95% confidence interval for the slope (Box 4.10). The standard error for the slope in Figure 4.3 is 0.153, so the 95% confidence interval is 1.4 to 2.0. We interpret this by saying that our best estimate of the **true** slope, the amount blood pressure increases with each year of age, is 1.7 and we are 95% confident that the true value lies somewhere between 1.4 and 2.0. This also implies that our best

Box 4.10

Regression coefficient, *b*, is the slope of the linear regression line
  b is the amount that *y* changes for a change of 1 unit of *x*

Confidence interval for a slope *b* (observed regression coefficient):
  95% CI for $b = b \pm 1.96 \times$ standard error of *b*

Box 4.11

| Quantifying the association between two factors (regression slope) No effect value = 0 | If p-value ≤0.05, observed slope is statistically significant. The true slope is unlikely to be 0; there is likely to be a real association |
| | If p-value >0.05, observed slope is not statistically significant. We do not have enough evidence to say that there is an association, i.e. that the true slope is not 0 |

estimate of how much blood pressure will increase every 10 years is 17 mmHg, and we are 95% confident that the true value lies between 14 mmHg and 20 mmHg.

If there was no association at all between age and systolic blood pressure then the line would be horizontal, and the slope would be 0; the **no effect value** for a regression coefficient. We can test to see whether the size of the regression coefficient is sufficiently large that it is unlikely to have arisen just by chance (Box 4.11). In the example the p-value for the regression coefficient is <0.001. This means that if there really were no association and the true slope is 0 (the no effect value), the likelihood of observing a slope as large as 1.7 (or greater) by chance alone is less than 1 in 1000. Therefore, there is only a very small chance that the true slope is 0. We can therefore say that there is an association between blood pressure and age.

The regression line can be used to predict the expected blood pressure for a man of a given age. For example, the estimated blood pressure of a man aged 55 is 164 mmHg ($71 + 1.7 \times 55$). This is the *average* blood pressure for a man aged 55, clearly there will be variation between the blood pressures of different men aged 55. Such predictions should only be made within the range of the values of age (x variable) on which the sample was based, here for men aged between 40 and 70 years. This is because although a straight line fits the data in this age range well, we might find that in younger or older men outside this range the relationship is different.

Blood pressure increases with age, so the slope of the line is upwards; the regression coefficient has a positive value. If a regression line slopes downwards this means that the value of one variable is decreasing as the other increases. Number of teeth decreases with age, so the slope of a regression line showing the association between number of teeth and age would slope downwards. The regression coefficient would have a negative value.

Correlation

How strong is the relationship between blood pressure and age? Suppose that if we knew someone's age we could predict their blood pressure exactly. Then all the points in our sample would lie on the regression line (Figure 4.5). In reality, we expect some

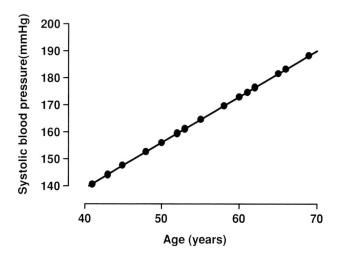

Figure 4.5 Scatter plot and fitted regression line of 15 men where there is a perfect relation between age and blood pressure.

scatter about the line. If there is very little scatter then there is a strong association between our two variables and we can use the line to make precise predictions. If the scatter is very wide, then there will only be a weak association between our variables and our predictions will be less precise. These are both illustrated in Figure 4.6.

The correlation coefficient summarises the strength of association between two variables, and takes values between 1 and −1 (Box 4.12). The correlation coefficient between systolic blood pressure and age (based on the data in Figure 4.2) is 0.89 which shows that the association is strong. Could this level of correlation be a chance finding in this particular study? We test to see whether the correlation coefficient is sufficiently large to make this unlikely, and obtain a p-value. Here the p-value is <0.001, so it is extremely unlikely that we would see an association as large as this purely by chance.

Box 4.12

Correlation coefficient, r, is a measure of the strength of association between two variables

r takes values between −1 and +1

$r = -1$ or $r = +1$ means that there is perfect correspondence between the two variables

$r = 0$ means there is no association between the two variables

A positive value of r means that when one variable increases, so does the other

A negative value of r means that when one variable increases the other decreases

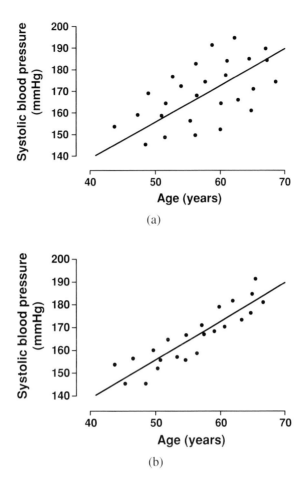

Figure 4.6 Scatter plots of age and blood pressure. Figure 4.6a shows a plot with a wide scatter and so the regression line is not useful for prediction. Figure 4.6b shows a plot with little scatter so the line would be good for prediction.

The square of the correlation coefficient, r^2, also gives us useful information (Box 4.13). It tells us how much of the variability in y is explained by x. The correlation coefficient between systolic blood pressure and age is 0.89, so $r^2 = 0.79$. This tells us that 79% of the variability in systolic blood pressure is explained by age.

Box 4.13

The correlation coefficient squared, r^2 is the amount of the variability in y-variable that is explained by the x-variable

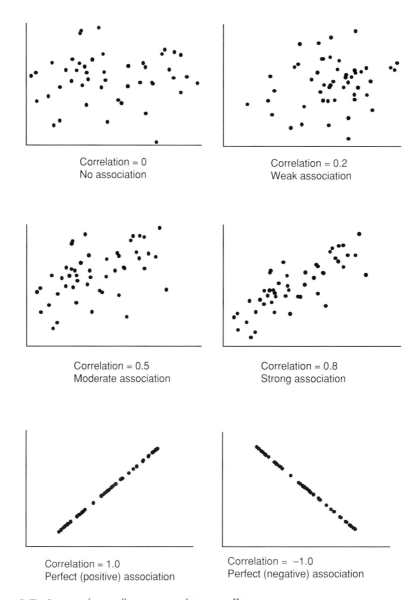

Figure 4.7 Scatter plots to illustrate correlation coefficients.

A correlation of 1 or −1 indicates that there is no scatter at all about the line and if we know the value of one of our two variables we could predict the other exactly. The sign in front of the correlation coefficient tells us whether the regression line is sloping up or down (the sign will be the same as that for the regression coefficient). A correlation of 0 means that there is no association between the two variables. Figure 4.7 shows scatter plots for data with different correlation coefficients.

Example of regression and correlation

Regression analyses are often performed on measurements from people, where each dot in the scatter plot represents an individual. They can also be applied to groups of people, where each dot represents a measurement for a group of individuals. If the group of people represents those living in a particular geographical area, this is called an ecological study. An example of this is presented from the following article, where each observation is based on a large number of children from an electoral ward.

Reference: Jones, C.M. and Worthington, H. Water fluoridation, poverty and tooth decay in 12-year-old children. *J Dent* 2000;28:389–393.

The abstract and Figure 4.8 are taken from the paper (see pp. 67.) In the study, the sampling unit was an electoral ward. For each ward the researchers had the following information:

- The Townsend score, a measure of social deprivation – the higher the score the greater the extent of social deprivation
- The mean number of DMFT (decayed, missing or filled teeth) for 12-year-old children in each ward (obtained from an NHS dental survey)
- Whether the water in the electoral ward was fluoridated

Figure 4.8 (p. 67) illustrates the regression of DMFT against Townsend score in two areas, non-fluoridated Liverpool and fluoridated Newcastle. There were 33 electoral wards in Liverpool and 26 in Newcastle. The two regression lines give us some idea of whether the relation between the state of children's teeth in a ward and the level of deprivation in that ward is similar in fluoridated and non-fluoridated areas.

The regression line for Liverpool, which is a non-fluoridated area, is:

$$\text{Mean ward DMFT} = 1.3496 + (0.1048 \times \text{Townsend score})$$

The regression coefficient is 0.1048, therefore, for every increase of one Townsend score unit (as poverty gets worse) the mean DMFT increases by 0.1048 (dental health gets worse). The p-value is again <0.05 indicating that the slope of the regression line is statistically significant, and the association is unlikely to be due to chance; the true slope is greater than 0. The correlation coefficient squared (here called R^2) is 0.49, indicating that 49% of the variation in the mean DMFT in different wards can be explained by the deprivation score. The correlation coefficient is 0.7, the square root of 0.49, indicating a fairly strong linear relation between Townsend score and mean DMFT.

The regression line for Newcastle, which is a fluoridated area, is:

$$\text{Mean ward DMFT} = 0.8433 + (0.0315 \times \text{Townsend score})$$

For every increase of 1 Townsend score unit the average mean DMFT in a ward increases by 0.0315. The p-value is again <0.05 indicating that the regression line is statistically significant. The proportion of variability explained by the regression line is 26%.

The slope of the regression line for non-fluoridated Liverpool (0.1048) is much steeper than that for fluoridated Newcastle (0.315). This implies that the relation between deprivation and tooth decay is stronger in areas where the water is not fluoridated. The authors went on to examine this in greater depth by performing a multiple linear regression, which looks at the effect of both deprivation and fluoridation jointly on DMFT. They concluded that 'the implementation of fluoridation markedly reduced tooth decay in 12-year-old children and that socio-economic dental health inequalities are reduced'.

To illustrate how large the effect of fluoridated water is, the authors looked at the value of the mean DMFT when the Townsend score was 0 (the average score for England):

$$\text{Mean DMFT for Liverpool is } (0.1048 \times 0) + 1.3496 = 1.3496$$

$$\text{Mean DMFT for Newcastle is } (0.0315 \times 0) + 0.8433 = 0.8433$$

$$\text{Percentage change from adding fluoride } [(1.3496 - 0.8433)/1.3496] \times 100 = 37\%$$

This means that when the deprivation score is set at the average for England, there is an estimated 37% reduction in the mean DMFT in 12-year-old children who live in fluoridated areas compared to those who do not.

Association and causation

In these examples of regression and correlation there are associations between blood pressure and age, and between social deprivation and dental health. *Finding an association between two factors does not mean that we can infer that one causes the other.* The association may be due to some other factor. For example, we know that blood pressure is associated with weight and that people put on weight as they get older. It is possible that all of the association between blood pressure and age could be due to older people being heavier. Weight **confounds** the association between blood pressure and age. The issues of causality and confounding are discussed in detail in Chapter 6.

Key points

Comparing two groups:

- Counting people: relative risk indicates how many times more likely a characteristic is in one group compared to another.
- Counting people: risk difference indicates how many more people in one group have the characteristic compared to another.
- Taking measurements on people: the difference between two means indicates how much larger, on average, the measurement is in one group than another.

Comparing two measurements taken from the same person or experimental unit:

- Linear regression quantifies the expected increase in one measurement when the other increases by 1 unit.

- A correlation coefficient quantifies the strength of the association between two measurements.
- An association between two factors does not mean that we can infer that one causes the other.

P-values and confidence intervals:

- P-values indicate whether the observed effect (relative risk, risk difference, correlation coefficient or regression slope) is likely to be a chance finding in a particular study or not.
- If the p-value ≤0.05, it is statistically significant and there is likely to be a true effect.
- If the p-value is >0.05, it is not statistically significant and there is insufficient evidence of a true effect.
- Confidence intervals provide a range within which the true effect is likely to lie.
- There is a relationship between p-values and confidence intervals.

ACKNOWLEDGEMENT

We are grateful to the *Journal of Dentistry* and the publishers, Elsevier, for kindly giving permission to reproduce the Abstract and Figure 1 of the paper by Jones and Worthington.

Exercise

1. Table 4.5 shows *hypothetical* relative risks for several risk factors for periodontitis. Express the relative risks as a percentage change in risk (i.e. excess risk or relative risk reduction). Interpret the results.
2. Table 4.6 shows the comparison's associated with whitening toothpastes and water. What can you say about Rembrandt versus Janina and Aquafresh Whitening versus water?
3. Table 4.7 shows the results of a regression analysis from a study based on all 5-year-old children in state schools in an area of London. In this study, there were 55 schools, and each school was associated with (i) a DMFT score for the children in the schools,

Table 4.5 Hypothetical relative risks for several risk factors of periodontitis.

Risk factor	Comparison	Relative risk
Vitamin C	High vs low vitamin C diet	0.35
Being male	Male vs female	0.80
Drinking tea	Tea drinker vs non-drinker	1.04
Dietary sugar	High vs low sugar consumption	1.39
Smoking	Current smoker vs never-smoker	5.50

Table 4.6 Comparison of selected whitening toothpastes (Sharif *et al.*, 2000).

Comparison of toothpastes (mean area of stain remaining after 5 minutes, optical density units) A vs B	Difference between the means Mean A − Mean B	95% CI for the difference	p-value
Rembrandt (78.0) vs Janina (65.7)	12.3	−0.06 to 24.6	0.051
Aquafresh Whitening (14.9) vs water (71.5)	−56.6	−72.4 to −40.8	<0.0001

(ii) the results of various test scores (mathematics score, English score, literacy test score) and (iii) a measure of social deprivation in the school geographical area (the Jarman score; high score = high level of deprivation). The proportion of children who had free school meals was also obtained from each school. (Reference: Muirhead, V. and Marcenes, W. An ecological study of caries experience, school performance and material deprivation in 5-year-old state primary school children. *Community Dent Oral Epidemiol* 2004; **32**:265–270). Several linear regression analyses were performed on the form:

$$\text{DMFT score} = a + b \times \text{explanatory variable}$$

The explanatory variables considered were: mathematics score, English score, literacy score, Jarman score, percentage of children who had free school meals. The regression coefficients are shown in Table 4.7.

(a) Which factors had a statistically significant association with DMFT?
(b) Interpret the regression coefficients and their confidence intervals.
(c) By how much does the DMFT score change if the mathematics score decreases by 5 units?
(d) What are the correlation coefficients for each factor? Which factor appears to have the strongest relationship with DMFT?

Answers on pp. 211–212

Table 4.7 Results of a linear regression analysis looking at the association between caries and specified factors.

Factor	Regression coefficient (*b*)	95% confidence interval	R^2 value
Mathematics	−0.16	−0.20 to −0.06	0.17
English	−0.13	−0.21 to −0.06	0.20
Literacy	−0.048	−0.072 to −0.024	0.23
Social deprivation (Jarman score)	0.021	0.003 to 0.039	0.095
% of children who have free meals	0.016	0.01 to 0.023	0.32

Journal of Dentistry 28 (2000) 389–393

www.elsevier.com/locate/jdent

Water fluoridation, poverty and tooth decay in 12-year-old children

C.M. Jones[a,*], H. Worthington[b]

[a]*Highland Health Board, Assynt House, Beechwood Park, Inverness IV2 3HG, UK*
[b]*Senior Lecturer in Dental Statistics, Department of Oral Health &. Development, Turner Dental School, University Dental Hospital of Manchester, Manchester M15 6FH, UK*

Received 9 July 1999; received in revised form 15 November 1999; accepted 10 December 1999

Abstract

Aim: To examine the influence of water fluoridation, and socio-economic deprivation on tooth decay in the permanent dentition of 12 year old children.

Setting: The North of England, fluoridated Newcastle and non-fluoridated Liverpool, A total of 6,638 children were examined.

Outcome Measures: Multiple Regression analysis of fluoride status, mean electoral ward DMFT in 1992/93 and ward Townsend Scores from the 1991 census.

Results: Social deprivation and tooth decay were significantly correlated in areas with and without water fluoridation. Multiple linear regression showed a statistically significant interaction between ward Townsend score, mean DMFT and water fluoridation, showing that the more deprived the area the greater the reduction in tooth decay.

At a Townsend score of zero (the English average) there was a predicted 37% reduction in decay in 12-year-olds in fluoridated wards.

Conclusions: Tooth decay is strongly associated with social deprivation. The findings confirm that the implementation of water fluoridation has markedly reduced tooth decay in 12-year-old children and that socio-economic dental health inequalities are reduced. ©2000 Published by Elsevier Science Ltd. All rights reserved.

Keywords: Water fluoridation; Deprivation; Townsend; Tooth decay; DMFT; Children; Electoral wards

C.M. Jones, H. Worthington Journal of Dentistry 28 (2000) 389–393

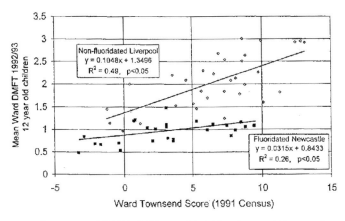

Mean Ward DMFT by Townsend score, fluoridated and non-fluoridated, with best-fit regression lines

Figure 4.8 Scattergram of mean ward DMFT of 12-year-old children by ward Townsend score, fluoridated and non-fluoridated, with best-fit regression lines.

Assessing the effectiveness of treatments

Perhaps the most important use of evidence-based dentistry is to be able to determine whether a treatment or preventive regimen actually works. Dental practitioners are contacted regularly by dental company representatives and may often see published papers in dental journals reporting on a new treatment or material. Such new therapies could involve dental materials, drugs, clinical techniques or any other method designed to prevent oral disease from occurring or to treat patients with existing disease.

Determining whether it would be worthwhile to use the new treatment on your own patients depends on understanding the evidence and its implications. For example, when the antibiotic metronidazole was first introduced for the treatment of acute ulcerative gingivitis, it would not have been sufficient just to say that 'metronidazole is effective' or 'metronidazole is very effective'. Both statements provide only a subjective judgement and are not sufficiently clear. What does 'effective' actually mean? Is it the percentage reduction in the *number of ulcerated interdental papillae* after, say, 7 days; or the *number of patients* who fully recover; or some other measure? Do the results of the effectiveness of metronidazole reflect a real effect of the drug or could they just be due to chance? How can we be sure that the beneficial effect seen in a particular study was not a fluke?

Clinical trials are almost always the best way of assessing a new treatment or preventive regimen. They are an experiment on humans, in which some people are given one treatment and some another treatment, so the effects of the two can be compared. New treatments are rarely accepted into routine dental practice until there is good evidence from one or more clinical trials.

This chapter introduces the scientific aspects of clinical trials – why they are useful and how to interpret the results. Most published papers present several different results on various aspects of the effects of treatment. When reading a paper on a clinical trial it is useful to bear in mind the aim of the study, the main outcome measure and the treatments given. This helps to focus on the relevant results and how they should be interpreted. Two clinical trials will be presented here, each using a different measure of effectiveness: one is based on counting people (to follow on from Chapter 2) and the other is based on taking measurements on people (to follow on from Chapter 3). The principles of design are similar in both trials, but the interpretation of the results depends on the measure of effectiveness used so the trials will be presented separately.

MAIN DESIGN ELEMENTS OF RANDOMISED CLINICAL TRIALS

Randomised trials provide the strongest evidence on the effectiveness of treatments. Their strength comes from four design elements: randomisation, blinding, control and specification of which patients are to be included. The study population in a clinical trial is defined by the inclusion and exclusion criteria. Because these concepts are central to all trials, we discuss them briefly before presenting the two examples.

Randomisation

Randomisation determines how subjects are allocated to treatments. Where two or more treatments are being compared, a decision has to be made about which treatment each patient will receive. If the choice of treatment is left to the researcher or patient, then patients with a certain characteristic, for example older patients or those with more severe disease, could be over-represented in one of the treatment groups. This will produce a **bias**, which affects the comparison of results between the groups. Randomisation involves assigning each subject to one of the treatments such that neither the researcher nor the patient is able to influence which treatment is received. The process of randomisation ensures that each individual entered in the trial has the same chance of being allocated to any treatment arm (Box 5.1).

The randomisation process itself is often performed by computer, which allocates a new patient to one of the treatment groups by doing the computing equivalent of tossing a coin. If the computer coin toss comes up heads the patient gets treatment A, and if it comes up tails the patient gets treatment B. Randomisation is designed to produce groups with similar characteristics. The characteristics of patients in different treatment groups will never be exactly the same; there will always be small differences in some attributes, such as age, sex or severity of illness, that arise just by chance. However randomisation aims to ensure that the only *systematic* differences between the arms of the trial are the treatments themselves. This means that any differences in outcome that we find at the end of the trial should be attributable to the treatment and not to any other factor.

Box 5.1

The objective of randomisation is to produce treatment groups that are as similar as possible with regard to characteristics other than treatment, so the only systematic difference between the two arms is the treatment given. Because of this, any differences in the results observed at the end of the trial should be due to the effect of the treatment and not to any other factors

The *person entering the patient* should not be able to predict the next treatment allocation

Blinding

If either the patient, or the clinician giving the treatment, or the researcher making the assessment of the outcome of treatment know which treatment has been given, this may adversely affect the results of the trial. Clinical trials are described as **double-blind** if neither the patient nor anyone involved in giving the treatment or assessing the patient is aware of the treatments given. In **single-blind** trials usually only the patient is blind to the treatment they have received. Patients or clinicians may have expectations associated with a particular treatment, and knowing which treatments were given can produce **bias**. Blinding removes this potential bias.

To understand how the lack of blinding can adversely affect the results, consider yourself to be the patient and then the dentist in a trial comparing an active drug with a placebo (an inactive drug). If, as a patient, you knew you were given an inactive substance this might affect how you respond to treatment. Similarly, if the dentist knew the patient was given the active treatment he or she might manage this patient differently from a patient given the inactive treatment. Either of these could result in patients on the active treatment appearing to do better than patients on the inactive treatment. This would bias the results in favour of the active treatment. Blinding, therefore, serves the useful function of removing patients' and clinicians' expectations that could influence the outcome of a trial and create an imbalance between the arms which is not due to the therapeutic properties of the active treatment.

Sometimes it is not possible to blind either the patient or the researcher. In such cases, we should have an outcome measure that does not depend on the opinions of the patient or researcher. For example, if we were to compare the effect of routine scaling and polishing with the effect of not scaling and polishing, then an assessment of plaque score made a year later during a clinical examination would be less prone to bias than a questionnaire on patient satisfaction.

Controlled trial

This simply means that there is a comparison group: the outcome of the patients on the new treatment is compared with that in a **control** group which is not receiving the new treatment. The control group usually receives either a placebo or the current standard of treatment. A placebo is a substance or procedure that has no known active component. Placebo is given rather than no treatment for the same reason that blinding is used. It avoids the possibility that the patient's expectations about how effective their treatment will be might bias the comparison between the two arms of the trial. When a standard treatment exists, it is unethical to give a placebo because this would deprive the patient of a possible health benefit.

Inclusion and exclusion criteria

The study population in a clinical trial is defined by a set of criteria which each patient has to fulfil to be entered in the trial. These criteria will always include the age range. Every trial will have its own set of criteria depending on the study question. Deciding who to include requires balancing the advantages of having a highly selected group against the advantages of including a wide variety of patients. A highly selected group is likely to respond to treatment in a similar manner, which may make it easier to demonstrate an effect of treatment. However, the results of the trial may then only apply to a small group of patients. A trial that includes a wide variety of patients will have more general application, but may have to be large to show that the treatment is effective across a range of people or conditions. Inclusion and exclusion criteria should have unambiguous and exact definitions so that the study population is precisely defined.

A CLINICAL TRIAL BASED ON COUNTING PEOPLE

Please read the paper reproduced on pp. 101–111 before continuing.

Reference: Averley, P.A., Girdler, N.M., Bond, S., Steen, N. and Steele, J. A randomised controlled trial of paediatric conscious sedation for dental treatment using intravenous midazolam combined with inhaled nitrous oxide or nitrous oxide/sevoflurane. *Anaesthesia* 2004;**59**:844–852.

What is the specific aim of the study?

The background section of this trial summarises the topic clearly. Performing dental surgery on anxious children can be difficult in general practice. General anaesthetic has been judged not to be sufficiently safe in a non-hospital setting (*paragraph 2*), so there is a need for an alternative method that is both safe and effective to allow the dentist to deliver the dental treatment successfully. The investigators provide a brief summary of possible alternatives, namely two sedative gases, nitrous oxide (*paragraph 1*) and sevoflurane (*paragraph 7*), and an intravenous sedative called midazolam (*paragraphs 5 and 6*). The aim is to investigate whether the addition of an analgesic gas to midazolam is effective or not. Nitrous oxide, as well as being a mild sedative gas and analgesic, also acts as a carrier gas for more potent gases such as sevoflurane, which might explain why there was no treatment arm with sevoflurane on its own.

Although the trial is based on a *sample* of children we want to describe the effect in *all* anxious children (the population of interest), not just the ones in the trial.

What is the intervention?

There are three interventions: Medical air, Nitrous oxide and Nitrous oxide plus sevoflurane. Each of these is followed by midazolam injected intravenously. It is useful to summarise the main aim of the trial, the treatments tested and main outcome measure as shown in Box 5.2. Details of the treatments are given in *paragraph 18*.

Box 5.2

What is the main aim of the trial?
When used with midazolam, is nitrous oxide with or without sevoflurane effective in sedating anxious children who are about to receive dental treatment?

What gas treatments are allocated to patients?
All children receive intravenous midazolam after inhaling one of three gases:
- Medical air
- Nitrous oxide
- Nitrous oxide plus sevoflurane

What is the main outcome measure?
Whether the dentist is able to complete dental treatment or not

What is the main outcome measure?

The main measure of efficacy is whether the dentist was able to complete the planned dental treatment or not (*paragraphs 9 and 30*). Is this outcome appropriate to address the aim of study to be addressed? There are other outcome measures available, for example, successful cannulation (to allow midazolam to be delivered) and level of anxiety (see first column of *Table 2* in the paper). Are any of these more appropriate than the one chosen or are there alternative measures that were not considered by the researchers? The main outcome measure needs to be clinically relevant. The children were attending for dental treatment, therefore what ultimately matters is whether this treatment could be delivered or not. Measuring anxiety levels is useful, but even if children become less anxious after being given a sedative gas they may still not want to go through with the dental treatment, so this would not be the best marker of efficacy. The main outcome measure chosen by the researchers is the most appropriate.

What is the study population?

Table 5.1 summarises the criteria on which children were included or excluded from the trial. The criteria involving assessment of the child's level of anxiety and co-operation were both based on established measurement tools. The invasiveness of treatment was assessed using a clearly defined scoring procedure (*paragraph 13*). The only criterion which relied solely on the judgement of the dentist was the child's degree of comprehension and understanding of the treatment. The criteria were broad enough to allow the results of the trial to be generalised to most children with moderate anxiety about having dental treatment.

Table 5.1 Inclusion and exclusion criteria for the trial by Averley *et al.* (2004).

Inclusion criteria	Age 6–14 years
	Referred by their dentist to QAMC (the specialist centre) for dental treatment using anxiety management
	Child's self-expressed level of anxiety 4 or more on a 10-point scale
	Dentist's assessment of child's co-operation scored 3 or more on a 6-point co-operation scale
	Invasiveness of the planned dental procedure (on a specified scale)
	Adequate degree of comprehension and understanding of treatment
	Acceptance of topical cream applied to hand and nasal hood
Exclusion criteria	History of hypersensitivity to benzodiazepines, sevoflurane, nitrous oxide or local anaesthetics

How was the study conducted?

This was a double-blind, controlled randomised trial, even though this phrase was not explicitly used in the paper.

Randomisation

The allocation to gas treatment group was co-ordinated by a nurse who was not involved in the trial (*paragraph 16*), an extra precaution to ensure that no one participating in the trial could influence allocation. The anaesthetist was informed of the allocated intervention prior to the appointment. Because the children were randomised in this way neither the child nor the dentist were able to decide which treatment was given. This would avoid biases such as the treating dentist giving the active gas to children who seemed more anxious, or severely anxious children refusing to have medical air – either of which could mean that severely anxious children would be under-represented in one of the arms.

Table 1 in the paper shows some of the characteristics of the children measured before they received treatment (called **baseline** characteristics); this allows us to assess whether randomisation produced similar intervention arms or not. All clinical trial reports should include a table like this to indicate whether there are differences, other than treatments, between the trial arms that might affect the comparison. The authors selected various factors that might influence whether children complete dental treatment or not and presented them according to each intervention group.

Most factors were evenly balanced between the groups, but the authors reported some differences in gender and in anxiety level. The data in *Table 1* show that there is a lower percentage of males among children who received nitrous oxide plus sevoflurane than among those who received air or nitrous oxide alone. This could only affect the results if males are more (or less) likely than females to complete their dental treatment. Similarly, children who received medical air have anxiety levels that are, on average, lower than the other two groups, and this could bias the results if these children were more likely to complete dental treatment (the effect of the sedative gases would be under-estimated). We therefore need to consider the extent to which the outcome of the trial could be affected by these imbalances. How much does it matter that some of the factors differ between the groups? The information in *Table 1* enables us to look at how much the differences might influence the results. For gender, the percentage of males in the nitrous oxide plus sevoflurane group is only 8–11 percentage points lower than in the other groups. The average anxiety level in the group receiving air is only about 0.5 lower than in groups 2 and 3 (a small difference given that anxiety is measured on a 10-point scale). It is, therefore, unlikely that differences of this size would materially affect the results.

Although the authors reported p-values for the differences between the groups (*Table 1* in the paper), it is the size of the imbalances that we need to consider rather than their statistical significance. The p-value tells us only whether an observed difference is likely to be due to chance. When the numbers of patients in the groups are very large, even small and unimportant differences in measured characteristics will be statistically significant. What matters is whether the differences are large enough to distort the main results.

Blinding

Both the dentist and the child were blind to the intervention given (*paragraph 19*). If the dentist knew that the child had received placebo (medical air) he or she might be more hesitant about completing dental treatment. Alternatively, if the dentist knew that the child had received one of the active gases, he or she might be more likely to attempt to complete dental treatment believing that the child had been adequately sedated. The authors mentioned that sevoflurane has a sweet odour (*paragraph 7*). If either the dentist or the child detected this as being different from air or the other gases they may not strictly have been blind to the intervention.

Controlled trial

The control arm was given medical air plus midozalom. This is ethically acceptable because there is no active gas that is routinely given in practice as a sedative, so the child was not being deprived of a beneficial standard therapy.

Sample size

Of the 2348 children assessed for eligibility, 848 were randomised to one of the three gas groups and 697 were included in the analysis (*Figure 1* in the paper). Usually, intervention arms have a similar number of patients, but in this trial there were fewer children in the group given medical air. This was because an early analysis of the results showed that children given air had a high failure rate, so recruitment to this group was stopped (*paragraph 29*).

What are the main results?

There are three main comparisons:

- Nitrous oxide versus air
- Nitrous oxide plus sevoflurane versus air
- Nitrous oxide plus sevoflurane versus nitrous oxide

The first two allow an assessment of whether the sedative gases confer a benefit over air. The third allows an assessment of whether adding sevoflurane to nitrous oxide is better than nitrous oxide alone.

The main results are conveniently summarised in *Table 2* in the paper. Columns 2 to 4 give the summary measure for the specified outcome measure in each gas group separately. Depending on the nature of the outcome the summary measure is presented as a percentage (where the outcome involves counting people) or a mean and standard deviation (where the outcome involves taking measurements on people, for example total dose of midazolam). The fifth column shows a statistical test to see if there are any differences between the three groups. If the test showed a difference between any of the three groups, then comparisons were made between each pair of gases to see where the difference lay. Columns 6–8 give the effect sizes associated with any pair of groups, together with their confidence intervals. Where the outcome is a count the comparison is expressed as a **relative risk**, and where the outcome is a mean the comparison is expressed as the difference in means.

The primary outcome of the trial, whether the dentist was able to complete the dental treatment or not, is displayed in the first row. The relative risks associated with this outcome are described in the next section, together with alternative ways of expressing these results. The relative risk was introduced in Chapter 2 and can be worked out easily from the numbers provided (Box 5.3).

Box 5.3

Group 1: The risk of successful completion of treatment = 94/174 = 0.5402
About half of the children in group 1 complete treatment

Group 3: The risk of successful completion of treatment = 249/267 = 0.9326
About nine-tenths of the children in group 3 complete treatment

Relative risk: How many times more likely is a child in group 3 to complete treatment than a child in group 1?

Relative risk = risk in group 3 ÷ risk in group 1 = 0.9326 ÷ 0.5402 = 1.73
A child in group 3 is 1.73 times as likely to complete treatment as a child in group 1.

Table 5.2 shows how the main results were calculated, along with a brief interpretation. For example, the comparison of nitrous oxide plus sevoflurane with air yields a

Table 5.2 The main comparisons of treatment groups in the trial by Averley *et al.* (2004).

Comparison (group 1 vs group 2)	Risk in group 1 R1	Risk in group 2 R2	Relative risk* R1 ÷ R2	Interpretation
Nitrous oxide vs air	204/256 (80%)	94/174 (54%)	1.47	Children given nitrous oxide are 1.47 times more likely to complete their treatment compared to those given air
Nitrous oxide plus sevoflurane vs air	249/267 (93%)	94/174 (54%)	1.73	Children given nitrous oxide plus sevoflurane are 1.73 times more likely to complete their treatment compared to those given air
Nitrous oxide plus sevoflurane vs nitrous oxide	249/267 (93%)	204/256 (80%)	1.17	Children given nitrous oxide plus sevoflurane are 1.17 times more likely to complete their treatment compared to those given nitrous oxide alone

* If two treatments had the same effect the ratio of the percentages would equal 1; the **no effect** value. The percentages R1 and R2 have been rounded.

relative risk of 1.73, showing that children given the combination of the two seda-tive gases are much more likely to complete dental treatment than those given air (1.73 times as likely). In Chapter 4 we showed alternative ways of interpreting rela-tive risks. For example, a relative risk of 1.73 also means that the risk of completing dental treatment is 73% greater among children given nitrous oxide plus sevoflurane compared to those given medical air (excess risk of 73%). These results indicate that the sedative gases were associated with an increase in the number of children for whom the dental treatment could be completed, and the combination of the two gases had a greater effect than nitrous oxide alone.

The implications of conducting a study based on a sample of people

Confidence intervals

We know that in the sample of children in the trial there was a beneficial effect of the sedative gases. But what we are really interested in is the effect of the sedative gases in *all* anxious children, not just the sample of children in the trial. How certain are we that in another group of children the relative risk of nitrous oxide versus air will be close to 1.47? We are unlikely to get an estimate of exactly 1.47 in a second sample of children, but could the true relative risk be equal to 1, indicating no effect? The **true effect** could only be determined by having a trial of every anxious child

Box 5.4

LARGE → Small → Narrow → PRECISE → FIRM
trial   standard error   95% CI   estimate of the effect   conclusions

Small → LARGE → WIDE → Imprecise → No
trial   standard error   95% CI   estimate   firm conclusions

now and in the future, which is clearly impossible. Although we can never measure this *exactly* we can use a 95% **confidence interval** to provide us with a *range* of likely true effect sizes.

The relative risk associated with nitrous oxide versus air is 1.47, with a 95% confidence interval of 1.27 to 1.72 (*Table 2* in the paper). We say that our best estimate of the **true effect** is 1.47 but we are 95% sure that whatever the actual value of the true effect is, it is likely to be in the range of 1.27 to 1.72. Therefore, the lowest the true relative risk is likely to be is 1.27 and the highest is 1.72. We are trying to decide whether the treatments (i.e. the gases) have the same effect or different effects. If they were the same the relative risk would take the value 1, the **no effect value**. Because the 95% CI for the relative risk does not include one, this is evidence against there being no effect of nitrous oxide compared with air.

The width of the confidence interval depends on the standard error, which itself depends on the size of the study (Box 5.4). When the study is very large the confidence interval will be narrow and it is likely that the true value lies within this narrow range. Table 5.3 shows what would happen to confidence intervals if we had found exactly the same results in a study ten times as large as this one, in a study 100 times as large, or a study one-tenth as large.

Although the estimate of the relative risk remains the same, as the study size increases the standard error gets smaller so the width of the confidence interval becomes narrower; we become more certain where the true value is likely to lie. In the very large study the true relative risk is likely to lie within a narrow range from 1.45 to 1.50. For a study one-tenth the size of that by Averley *et al.* the confidence interval includes 1, the no effect value. This confidence interval tells us that based on this small trial the true relative risk could be as low as 0.88 (a risk decrease) or as high

Table 5.3 The 95% confidence interval for studies of different sizes but with the same estimate of relative risk.

	Risk on nitrous oxide	Risk on medical air	Relative risk	Confidence interval
Study 1/10 as big	20/26	9/17	1.45*	0.88 to 2.38
Averley study	204/256	94/174	1.47	1.27 to 1.72
Study 10 times as big	2040/2560	940/1740	1.47	1.41 to 1.55
Study 100 times as big	20400/25600	9400/17400	1.47	1.45 to 1.50

* This is the closest to 1.47 that we can get with a study that is 1/10 as large.

as 2.38 (a large risk increase). Therefore the effect could be either in favour of air or in favour of nitrous oxide, or no effect at all (because the confidence interval includes 1). For our study and the larger ones the confidence interval does not contain 1, both the lower and upper ends of the confidence interval are greater than 1 and the values within that range are all in favour of nitrous oxide.

When interpreting the results both the relative risk (1.47) and its confidence interval (1.27 to 1.72) are needed to answer the following questions:

- How large is the effect?
- Does the confidence interval contain the no effect value of 1?
- What are the lowest and highest values that the true relative risk is likely to take?

Alternative ways of describing the effectiveness of a treatment

The relative risk tells us how many *times more* (or less) effective the treatment gas is in one group compared to another. But it does not indicate the *number* of patients who would benefit. There are two commonly used measures that do this: the **risk difference** (which was discussed in Chapters 2 and 4) and the **number needed to treat**. These two measures were not presented in the paper but they can be calculated using the results in *Table 2*.

The **risk difference** is simple to obtain. The relative risk for each comparison is the *ratio* of two proportions (Table 5.2). The risk difference is obtained by *subtracting* one proportion from the other. If two treatments had the same effect the difference between the proportions would equal 0, therefore a risk difference of 0 would indicate no effect. Table 5.4 shows the risk differences and number needed to treat for each of the three main comparisons. For the comparison of nitrous oxide versus air the risk difference is 26% (80 − 54). This means that for every 100 children treated with nitrous oxide there would be an *extra 26* who would complete their treatment compared to a group of 100 who had been given air. The **number needed to treat** quantifies how many patients have to be given a new therapy so that one extra patient can benefit,

Table 5.4 Risk difference and number needed to treat for the main comparisons in the trial by Averley *et al.* (2004).

Comparison (1 vs group 2)	Risk in group 1 R1	Risk in group 2 R2	Risk difference, %[*] R1 − R2 (95% CI)	Number needed to treat[*] 100/(R1 − R2) (95% CI)
Nitrous oxide vs air	204/256 (80%)	94/174 (54%)	26 (17 to 34)	4 (3 to 6)
Nitrous oxide plus sevoflurane vs air	249/267 (93%)	94/174 (54%)	39 (31 to 47)	3 (2 to 3)
Nitrous oxide plus sevoflurane nitrous oxide	249/267 (93%)	204/256 (80%)	13 (8 to 19)	8 (5 to 12)

[*] Rounded to nearest whole number.

compared to giving another therapy. We can find the number needed to treat from the risk difference.

Outcome: successful completion of dental treatment
Group A (nitrous oxide): risk $P_A = 204/256 = 0.80$
Group B (air): risk $P_B = 94/174 = 0.54$

$$\text{Number needed to treat (NNT): } \frac{1}{P_A - P_B} = \frac{1}{0.80 - 0.54} \approx 4$$

An estimated 4 children need to be treated with nitrous oxide for 1 extra child to complete dental treatment, compared with children given air

The comparisons based on risk differences (Table 5.4) lead us to the same conclusions as those based on relative risks (Table 5.2), namely that the sedative gases are better than air. The 95% CIs for the risk differences do not include 0 (the no effect value when we are dealing with risk differences). This is consistent with the 95% CI for the relative risk not including 1 (the no effect value when we take the ratio of two risks).

Relative risk or risk difference?

Relative risks have the advantage of usually being independent of the prevalence of the risk factor and therefore applicable to populations other than the study population. For example, in the current trial 54% of children were able to complete their dental treatment when using air alone, but this increased by a factor of 1.47 when using nitrous oxide to 80% ($\approx$54% $\times$ relative risk of 1.47). In another population where only 20% would normally complete treatment in the absence of a sedative gas, one would expect this also to increase by a factor of 1.47, that is to 29% (= 20% $\times$ 1.47). In other words, it is likely that the relative risk estimate of 1.47 will be applicable to other groups of children.

The risk difference, however, will vary in different populations depending on the prevalence, but it has an advantage over the relative risk in that it tells us *how many* people will benefit if we introduce a new treatment. In the example above the risk difference between nitrous oxide and air is 26% (80%–54%) which means that if 100 children are given the nitrous oxide we expect 26 more children to complete treatment than if they had been given air. In contrast, a population where the risk of completing dental treatment in children given air is 20% and the relative risk

Table 5.5 Risk of completing dental treatment: the effect of the change in the background prevalence (R1) on the relative risk and risk difference.

Risk in children given air R1	Risk in children given nitrous oxide R2	Relative risk R2 ÷ R1	Risk difference R2 − R1	Number needed to treat 100/(R2 − R1)
54.0%	79.7%	1.47	26%	4
20.0%	29.4%	1.47	9%	11

Box 5.5

Relative risk:

Usually constant across different populations and independent of the underlying prevalence (or incidence) of the disease of interest.
It is a measure of the treatment effect that is generalisable to different populations

Risk difference:

Depends on the underlying prevalence (or incidence) and so may vary from population to population.
It is a measure of the number of people that the treatment will affect in a particular population

is also 1.47, the risk difference between nitrous oxide and air is 9% (29%–20%). So in this population, if 100 children were given nitrous oxide we would expect only nine more children to complete treatment than if they had been given air (Table 5.5). Both relative risk and risk difference are useful ways of comparing counts of people, although the former is more often reported because it can be generalised directly to other patient populations (Box 5.5).

Is the observed effect a chance finding?

When looking at any research we need to consider whether the observed results are likely to represent a real effect in the population or are just a chance finding in the particular sample of people we have chosen. When we measure an outcome in two different groups of people, natural variation will mean that the values in the two groups will never be identical. If the difference in outcome between the groups is very large then it is unlikely to be due to chance variation, whereas if it is small it may be due to chance. A **statistical test** gives us information on which we can base decisions about whether the result we find in a study is likely to be due to chance. A statistical test generates a p-value; this is defined as the probability of finding a difference as large, or larger than, the one in our sample just by chance, if there really is no underlying difference between the groups. In *Table 2* in the paper, there is a statistical test that compares the proportion of children completing dental treatment between the three groups; χ^2 (chi-squared) = 9.64, p <0.001. The figure of 9.64 is obtained by a mathematical formula incorporating the three percentages as well as the number of children in each treatment group. This is called a **test statistic** and it is used to produce the p-value. The test statistic itself and how it is derived is not of importance for the purpose of this discussion (for details see books on epidemiology and medical statistics in Further Reading); what matters is the interpretation of the p-value. In the study on sedation, if there really were no effect of either of the two sedative gases, the proportion of children completing dental treatment would be the same in all groups. However, there are clear differences between the groups (Table 2). The probability of seeing effects as large as these, when in fact there is no real difference, is less than 1 in 1000, summarised in the expression 'p <0.001'. So, effects of this magnitude are unlikely to be due to chance alone.

Box 5.6

BIG differences → small p-value → difference is unlikely to be due to chance
(we conclude there is a real effect)

Small differences → LARGE p-value → insufficient evidence to conclude there is a
real effect
(but we cannot say there is no effect)

By convention, the value of $p \leq 0.05$ is taken to be statistically significant. When $p = 0.05$ this tells us that in 1 of 20 studies of the same size we could expect to see an effect as large as the one we have found purely through chance. We need to be aware that there is always some possibility, however small, that any difference we find could be due to chance rather than a real underlying difference. The smaller the p-value the less likely that this would be the case (Box 5.6).

When a result is statistically significant we have evidence that the difference produced by our intervention is sufficiently large that it is unlikely to have arisen just by chance alone. If we get a result that is not statistically significant then we cannot conclude that there is no difference between our interventions. All we can say is that we have insufficient evidence to show a difference. There are several options we have to consider (Box 5.7). The size of a study is vitally important in determining whether it will be able to show a statistically significant difference. If you wanted to find out whether a drug reduced mortality from heart attack from 60% to 50% – a difference of 10% – it would be no use doing a study with only ten people in each group. You would then expect to see six deaths in one group and five in the other, a difference of only 1 death. This is not enough on which to base a firm conclusion. Such a study would not be large enough to detect a difference in mortality of 10%. There is a danger that a new therapy may be rejected as ineffective on the basis of a study that is too small to pick up a clinically important difference. Sample size will be discussed in more detail in Chapter 8.

As discussed in Chapter 4 there is a relationship between statistical significance and confidence intervals: if the confidence interval contains the no effect value, then the difference will not be statistically significant; if the confidence interval does not contain the no effect value then the difference will be statistically significant (Box 5.8). For example, in the comparison of successful completion of dental treatment between

Box 5.7

Why was the result not statistically significant? The possibilities are:

- There really is no difference
- There is a real difference, but by chance we picked a sample that did not show this
- There is a real difference but the study was too small to detect it

Box 5.8

Measure of efficacy	No effect value	Confidence interval	p-value
Relative risk	1	If 95% CI includes 1	Results are not statistically significant (p >0.05)
		If 95% CI excludes 1	Results are statistically significant (p ≤ 0.05)
Risk difference	0	If 95% CI includes 0	Results are not statistically significant (p >0.05)
		If 95% CI excludes 0	Results are statistically significant (p ≤ 0.05)

groups 2 and 1 (first row of *Table 2* in the paper) the relative risk is 1.47 and the confidence interval is 1.27 to 1.72. Because the confidence interval does not include 1 this tells us that the statistical test comparing these two groups would produce a p-value that is <0.05.

Clinical importance and statistical significance

The results of a trial need to be considered from two perspectives – **clinical importance** and **statistical significance**. Clinical importance involves considering the size of the treatment effect and deciding whether the effect is large enough to alter your current practice. Statistical significance is less subjective, it is determined by the p-value; the smaller the value the less likely the observed results are just due to chance. In the trial, the p-value associated with comparing the successful completion rate of the three gases was <0.001. This shows that the difference between the interventions is so large that it is unlikely to have occurred by chance alone.

Deciding whether a result is clinically important depends on looking further than just the p-value by considering the size of the treatment effect. If, for example, a study on diet and weight loss found that there was a statistically significant difference between two diets after 6 months, but the size of the difference in weight loss was only 0.5 kg, then you would probably not recommend one diet as being clinically better than the other. If the size of the difference were 5 kg, you would recommend the more effective diet. Clinical importance depends not only on finding that the groups differ, but also on just how large that difference is. In this study, comparing air with nitrous oxide plus sevoflurane yielded a risk difference of 39% with a confidence interval of 31% to 47%. This implies that if nitrous oxide plus sevoflurane is used rather than air, 39 more children in every 100 are likely to complete their treatment. It is likely that the smallest number of extra children who complete dental treatment is 31 and the largest number could be 47. Based on this evidence we would say that the use of nitrous oxide plus sevoflurane is likely to increase substantially the number of children who complete dental treatment and the increase is clinically important.

Both clinical importance and statistical significance should be considered when deciding whether to introduce a new treatment into practice. An example of how to balance clinical importance and statistical significance can be found in the paper where the authors reported results on successful cannulation (*paragraph 30*). Among the subgroup of children in whom cannulation was achieved, the odds ratio (interpreted in a similar way to relative risk) of completing dental treatment for those given nitrous oxide compared with those given air is 1.61, 95% confidence interval 0.96 to 2.72, p-value 0.075 (*paragraph 30*). Here, the confidence interval includes 1 implying that it is possible that the **true** relative risk indicates no difference between the two groups. This is consistent with the p-value (0.075) being just above 0.05; the increase in odds is not strictly statistically significant. If the interpretation of this result was based on the p-value alone, we could conclude that there was no evidence for an effect. However, the p-value has just missed significance (it is not far from 0.05) and most of the range of the confidence interval is above 1, indicating an effect that is in favour of nitrous oxide. In the whole sample nitrous oxide was effective, so it is plausible that it is also effective in the subgroup of children who were cannulated.

Important effects could be missed if decisions are based solely on statistical significance without looking at the effect size and the confidence interval. In a situation where the confidence interval indicates that there may be a clinically useful effect, but the study is too small to have the power to detect this, further research based on a larger sample may be useful.

Side effects and safety

In all clinical trials comparing treatment regimens it is important to report side effects (adverse events or reactions) if they have occurred. In trials using a drug it is a legal requirement to report serious side effects.

In dental trials side effects are relatively rare. Many trials, although large enough to yield statistically significant results associated with the main outcome, will not be sufficiently large to allow robust conclusions to be drawn on rare side effects. This is probably the case with the current trial (*paragraph 37*). The investigators report that the side effects were minor and the only ones that were clinically important were associated with vomiting. There were six cases of vomiting and all occurred in the nitrous oxide plus sevoflurane group, suggesting that they were caused by using several sedatives together (*paragraph 38*). We could calculate the **number needed to harm**, which has a similar interpretation to number needed to treat, but the outcome measure is associated with side effects.

Outcome (adverse effect): vomiting
Group A (nitrous oxide plus sevoflurane): risk $P_A = 6/267 = 0.022$
Group B (air): risk $P_B = 0/174 = 0$

$$\text{Number needed to harm (NNH):} \quad \frac{1}{P_A - P_B} = \frac{1}{0.022 - 0} = 44$$

An estimated 44 children need to be given nitrous oxide plus sevoflurane for 1 extra child to suffer vomiting compared with children given air.

Comparing the proportion of children who vomited using nitrous oxide plus sevoflurane (6/267) with nitrous oxide (0/256) produces a p-value of 0.03, and the p-value for the comparison with air (0/174) is 0.08 (the p-values were not reported in the paper but can be calculated from the proportions). Although these p-values are close to the cut-off for statistical significance (0.05), it would take a larger study to confirm that this was not just a chance effect. Because vomiting only occurred in 2% of children we can conclude that despite the possibility that side effects may be more common in one of the treatment groups, they are short term and infrequent; there is no cause for concern about them.

How good is the evidence?

In this section we consider several aspects of how the study was designed and how the data were analysed.

Trial design

This was a double-blind, randomised controlled trial. The randomisation process, blinding and control group all contribute to removing the potential biases associated with differences in characteristics between the gas treatment groups, preferences in treatments and human expectation.

Study size

Was the study large enough to enable meaningful comparisons to be made? A fundamental aspect of trial design is determining how many patients should be included. When a trial has too few patients it is difficult to detect clinically important effects, so the trial produces equivocal results. A larger trial is required to answer the research question satisfactorily. Large trials usually produce conclusive results and provide precise estimates of treatment effect. However, if they are too large, there will be patients who could have benefited from the treatment if the trial had finished earlier. It is more common to find trials that are too small to answer the question specified than trials that are too large.

The size of the current trial was large enough to produce unequivocal results that are clinically important. The calculation of the sample size (called power calculation) was based on results from a small pilot study (*paragraph 12*). We discuss sample size further in Chapter 8.

Compliance

In many trials there are some patients who do not take the allocated treatment as specified in the study protocol. These patients are called **non-compliers**. In trials where patients take a drug for a period of time there can be a difference in compliance between the treatment groups, which might be due to side effects of one of the drugs. When compliance is low, it is useful to try to determine the reasons for this. Even when the treatment is biologically effective, if few people are prepared to tolerate its side effects it may not be worthwhile offering it in practice.

In this study compliance can be assessed by looking at the proportion of children in each gas treatment arm who received their allocated gas and seeing if these are similar. The percentage of children who received their allocated gas was 78% in group 1 (air), 84% in group 2 (nitrous oxide) and 83% in group 3 (nitrous oxide and sevoflurane) (*Figure 1* in the paper). Non-compliers were excluded from the analyses in the paper. Re-analysing the data with the non-compliers included does not change the main result (see section below on 'Intention-to-treat analysis').

Lost to follow-up (or drop-outs)

When a patient is **lost to follow-up** it is not possible to obtain a measure of the main outcome, and such patients may have to be excluded from the analysis. In the current trial, the main outcome is whether the dentist was able to complete treatment, and this is known for every child. The problem of loss to follow-up usually occurs in trials where patients are expected to return to the dentist for assessment after a period of time. For example, in a trial of a new antibiotic to treat acute ulcerative gingivitis the main outcome could be determined one month after treatment. If, despite attempts to contact them, some patients do not return for their one-month appointment, we would be unable to say whether they have recovered or not. In this situation they are lost to follow-up. Investigators often make strenuous efforts to ensure that loss to follow-up is minimised and hope that it is similar between treatment arms. Baseline characteristics of subjects that are lost to follow-up are often reported in the published paper to show the reader that there are no substantial differences between the treatment groups in the types of patients who were not followed up.

Intention-to-treat analysis

Intention-to-treat is a fundamental approach to analysing data from clinical trials. Patients are analysed according to the treatment arm to which they were randomised, whether they actually received that treatment or not. This may seem to be an unfair method of comparing treatments. Why should someone be included in an analysis looking at the effect of a treatment if they have not received the treatment? The problem with leaving them out of the analysis is that the balance of patient characteristics achieved by randomisation could be lost. This is illustrated in the example shown in Figure 5.1 of a hypothetical trial of 100 patients with oral cancer randomised to receive either surgery or chemotherapy.

The (ten) inoperable patients are clearly different in some way from the other patients in the surgery group: they probably have a worse prognosis. Comparisons (A) and (B) will both be biased and favour surgery. In comparison (A) the ten inoperable patients have been taken out of the surgery group, but the equivalent ten inoperable patients in the chemotherapy group are still there. Comparison (B) makes things even more unbalanced between the groups by taking the inoperable patients from the surgery group and adding them to the chemotherapy group. The only fair comparison that we can make is (C). We cannot compare *pure surgery* versus *pure chemotherapy* in this trial. What we can compare is the treatment strategy of *surgery followed by chemotherapy if surgery is not possible* versus *chemotherapy*. Many trials are designed to make such comparisons.

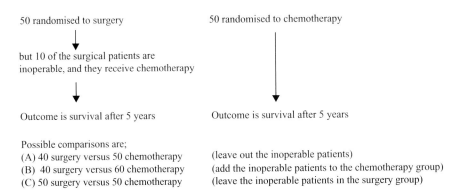

Figure 5.1 Hypothetical study of 100 patients with lung cancer who were randomised to receive surgery or chemotherapy.

The principle underlying intention-to-treat analysis is to retain the balance achieved by randomisation. It is possible that non-compliers differ from the rest of the patients in the study, so removing them from the analysis could also affect the balance of prognostic factors between the treatment groups. An analysis that includes only those patients who received their allocated treatment (compliers) is sometimes called a **per protocol** analysis (comparison (A) in Figure 5.1). In the trial on sedative gases, although the analyses were reported to be intention-to-treat (*paragraph 26*), they were in fact per protocol analyses. *Figure 1* in the paper states that some of the children assigned to the three groups were excluded from the analysis if they failed to attend, did not have EMLA cream applied or rejected the nose mask. The results presented in the paper are, therefore, based only on children who received the allocated treatments. This is similar to comparison (A) in the oral cancer example above (Figure 5.1). However, we know the results for these excluded children – none of them completed dental treatment at the time – so we can work out the risks with these children included by adding them to the denominator of the risk calculation. The results for an intention-to-treat analysis can be worked out from the information given in the paper, shown in Table 5.6. Fortunately in this case, the intention-to-treat results are similar to the per protocol results, so although the investigators reported the per protocol analysis this does not invalidate their conclusions. In some trials the results of the intention-to-treat analysis will be very different from the per protocol analysis. If a trial report does not present intention-to-treat analyses, it is worth trying to calculate them if possible.

Summary of trial design and analysis

Box 5.9 summarises the main design and analysis considerations. If these criteria are fulfilled this increases our confidence in the results of the trial. This trial was randomised, controlled and double-blind; a high proportion of children received their allocated treatment; and there were no losses to follow-up. The sample size was based on results from a pilot study and was large enough to detect clinically

Table 5.6 Relative risks and risk differences for per protocol analysis and intention to treat analysis (Averley *et al.*, 2004).

Group 1 vs Group 2	Per protocol analysis (as reported)				Intention-to-treat analysis			
	Group 1 R1	Group 2 R2	Relative risk R1/R2	Risk difference R1 − R2	Group 1 R1	Group 2 R2	Relative risk R1/R2	Risk difference R1 − R2
Nitrous oxide vs air	204/256	94/174	1.47	26%	204/306	94/222	1.57	24%
Nitrous oxide plus sevoflurane vs air	249/267	94/174	1.73	39%	249/320	94/222	1.84	35%
Nitrous oxide plus sevoflurane vs nitrous oxide	249/267	204/256	1.17	14%	249/320	204/306	1.17	11%

important differences. A possible weakness of the study was that the results were based on a per-protocol analysis. However, re-analysis on an intention-to-treat basis supported the results found in the per-protocol analysis. From this, it seems that the authors findings are well supported.

Box 5.9

Trial design	Was the study: randomised controlled blinded as far as possible	Yes Yes Yes
Compliance	Was compliance similar between the gas treatment arms? If not how might this affect the conclusions?	Yes
Lost to follow-up	Was follow-up similar between the gas treatment arms? If not, how might this affect the conclusions?	No follow-up required
Sample size	Was the study large enough to detect a clinically important effect?	Yes
Intention-to-treat analysis	Was the analysis on an intention-to-treat basis?	No, but an intention-to-treat analysis produces similar results

What does the study contribute to dental practice?

The main result was statistically significant, the size of the effect was clinically important, and we have confidence in the reliability of the trial results. The next step is to consider how the results of this trial should affect practice.

- Who will the results apply to: is this sample representative of the population of interest and can the findings be applied to other groups?
- Cost–benefit: Does the treatment have the potential to cause harm and if so do the benefits outweigh the harm?
- Financial cost-effectiveness: Is the benefit worth the financial cost of the treatment?

Who will the results apply to?

The population of interest in the study is children who are anxious about dental treatment. The children in the study had been referred to a single centre; would they be representative of anxious children elsewhere? The centre was large, with a wide catchment area and it is unlikely that children attending the centre would be affected by the gases in a different way from children attending specialist centres in other parts of the country.

If many of the children approached had refused to take part in the study, then the results may only be applicable to a highly selected group of children. In fact, only 117 of the children approached refused to take part (*Figure 1*), so the treatment gases should be acceptable to the majority of anxious children, not just to a highly selected group.

Can the findings be extended to other populations? The children had all been referred for anxiety management, so they had moderate to high levels of anxiety about receiving dental surgery. It is possible that children with lower levels of anxiety could also benefit from these gas treatments, but to be sure of this further research would be needed. Anxious adults might benefit too; again further research would be required to show this. Care is needed in deciding how far to extrapolate research findings to populations who have different characteristics from the subjects included in the trial.

Cost–benefit

The side effects of the drugs used in this study were minimal (a few cases of vomiting). The benefits were considerable, so they outweigh the possible harm. Some treatments in other areas of dentistry may have more severe side effects, so the balance between cost and benefit can be more difficult to determine.

Financial cost-effectiveness

The trial report does not give any details on the costs of using the various gases. However, if the alternative to a sedative gas is a general anaesthetic, use of the sedative gases is likely to be cheaper.

Summary

In summary, this was a well-conducted large study. It provides evidence that intravenous sedation (midazolam) in combination with inhaled gaseous agents is a more effective method of sedation for dental treatment of anxious children than midozalam alone. Nitrous oxide with sevoflurane is more effective than nitrous oxide on its own. Side effects were infrequent and short term. Dentists faced with children who are worried about having dental procedures could consider these methods as a safe and effective approach that will allow dental treatment to be delivered successfully in a primary care setting. This method of sedation is an alternative to general anaesthesia, which has to be performed in hospital. However, the combination of sedative agents needs anaesthetists and so this treatment needs to be conducted in specialist centres, similar to the one in the trial.

A CLINICAL TRIAL BASED ON TAKING MEASUREMENTS ON PEOPLE

The following is an example of a clinical trial in which the main outcomes were measurements taken on people, rather than counts of the number of people responding to treatment (as in the paper in the previous section).

Reference: Lao, L., Bergman, S., Hamilton, G.R., Langenberg, P. and Berman, B. Evaluation of acupuncture for pain control after oral surgery. A placebo-controlled trial. *Arch Otolaryngol Head Neck Surg* 1999;**125**:567–572.

Several concepts associated with randomised trials are similar to those already discussed for the trial of sedation in children, therefore we will only provide selected parts of this paper – the Abstract, the Patients and Methods and *Table 1* (see pp. 112–114). The main results have been extracted from the text and put in a table (see below).

What is the specific aim of the study?

The trial aims to determine whether acupuncture is associated with a reduction in pain compared with placebo in patients having oral surgery.

What is the main outcome measure?

The primary outcomes are associated with pain. Pain after oral surgery is expected and there are several aspects to it, including when the pain occurs (whether it is immediate or after the local anaesthetic has worn off) and what it is due to: swelling or bruising, jaw muscle spasm or dry socket, which could occur about 7–10 days later.

What sort of pain is acupuncture meant to prevent? Is the effect short or long term? Because acupuncture is delivered only once for 20 minutes it may be less likely to affect long-term pain. Experiencing immediate post-operative pain, about 2–3 hours later, is not unusual, so if acupuncture can prevent this or reduce the effect it would be a clinically useful technique.

Self-reported pain by the patient

This was assessed in several ways: (i) the length of time that elapsed after surgery before moderate pain was experienced, (ii) the length of time before asking for pain relief medication and (iii) the number of pain relief tablets taken after surgery during the first 24 hours and the first seven days (*paragraphs 3 and 4*). Both (i) and (ii) were assessed while the patient was still in the clinic (*paragraph 4*). Because the aim of the study was to evaluate pain relief these three measures are all clinically relevant. Also, they should not be affected by bias because the patients were blind to treatment.

What is the intervention?

Some patients received acupuncture and the others received placebo. Acupuncture involved inserting needles into four locations on the skin on the side of the face where the tooth was to be extracted (*paragraph* 2). The placebo involved placing the needles next to the same part of the skin, where one was taped in place but not inserted, and the area of the skin was tapped using a plastic needle and manipulated to give some sensation.

What is the study population?

Table 5.7 shows the criteria used in the trial to include or exclude patients (*paragraph 1*). These criteria are precise and easy to follow for dentists entering patients in the trial. The only criterion that is not precisely specified in the paper is 'Taking medications that might confound the results'. The medications are not listed in the paper, but it is likely that there was a list which was used when selecting patients for entry to the trial.

Table 5.7 Inclusion and exclusion criteria for the trial by Lao *et al.* (1999).

Inclusion criteria:	Age 18–40 years In good health (American Society of Anesthesiologists class I or II) Needs extraction of one mandibular (lower) partial bony impacted third molar No history of prior treatment with acupuncture
Exclusion criteria:	Presenting with any oral disease Taking medications that might confound the results History of bleeding diathesis History of allergy to the medication used in the study Women who were pregnant or lactating

Table 5.8 Demographic variables in the treatment and control groups (Lao *et al.*, 1999).*

Variable	Acupuncture group (n = 19)	Control group (n = 20)
Sex		
Male	11 (58)	11 (55)
Female	8 (42)	9 (45)
Race		
Asian	1 (5)	0 (0)
Black	1 (5)	2 (10)
Hispanic	2 (11)	1 (5)
White	15 (79)	17 (85)
Age, years		
18–22	8 (42)	8 (40)
23–27	7 (37)	10 (50)
28–34	4 (21)	1 (10)

* Mean (standard deviation) age for the acupuncture group was 23.4 (4.7) years and for the control group it was 24.0 (3.8) years.

How was the study conducted?

Randomisation

This was a randomised trial of 39 patients, therefore neither the patient nor the oral surgeon or acupuncturist was able to affect whether a patient received acupuncture or placebo (*paragraph 2*). The randomisation should reduce or remove the effect of any possible biases which would lead to systematic differences between the groups. Table 5.8 (*Table 1* in the paper) shows that randomisation worked, in that it produced two groups with similar characteristics.

Placebo-controlled

The researchers provided a placebo treatment in which the same procedure was followed as for the acupuncture group with the exception that the needles were not actually inserted (*paragraph 2*).

Blinding

The trial was double-blind because both the patient and dentist were unaware which intervention was given. Clearly, it was not possible to blind the acupuncturist. To ensure that the patients were not able to guess which treatment they received their eyes were covered during the operation and tapping applied within the mouth (*paragraph 2*). In this trial it was particularly important for the patient to be blind because the two of the main outcomes were subjective (length of time pain-free after surgery and time taken to ask for pain relief medication), both of which relied completely on the patient's self-assessment. If patients were aware of their treatment this could introduce bias: a patient who knew he or she had acupuncture might wait longer to ask for medication thinking the acupuncture should have worked, while a patient who knew they were given placebo might wait less time because they were aware that they had not been given an 'active' treatment. Differences between the groups in the average time they waited before seeking pain relief could then be due to their knowledge of whether they had been given an active treatment or not, rather than to any biological effect of the acupuncture. This could lead to the conclusion that acupuncture was better that placebo, when in fact it was not. Although the acupuncturist was not blind this is of less concern because the surgery was performed by the dental surgeon and the outcome measures were reported by the patient.

Non-compliers

There were none here. The treatment was given once and all patients had either acupuncture or placebo.

Lost to follow-up (drop-outs)

There were none for those outcomes assessed while the patient was still in the dental surgery (e.g. time taken to ask for medication). There may have been drop-outs for pain assessment at 24 hours and at 7 days (i.e. patients may not have completed the pain questionnaires at these times) but this was not specified in the paper.

Intention-to-treat analysis

The analysis was performed on the basis of intention-to-treat.

What are the main results?

The results for this trial were given in the main text of the paper. For convenience they are summarised in Table 5.9. The results are interpreted below (numbers from the table have been rounded to the nearest integer).

Time without pain after surgery

Patients given acupuncture had a longer period of time without pain after surgery compared with those given placebo. The difference in the means shows that they were free of pain, on average, for an extra 79 minutes. This is a large difference that is clinically worthwhile. The difference was statistically significant ($p = 0.01$) so this large difference is unlikely to be due to chance. The 95% confidence interval provides a range of likely values for the true effect of acupuncture compared to placebo. The true extra pain-free time could be as low as 18 minutes or as great as 140 minutes.

Time before asking for pain medication after surgery

Patients given acupuncture were able to wait longer before asking for pain relief medication compared with those given placebo. They waited, on average, a further 76 minutes. This too is a large difference that is clinically worthwhile, and again the

Table 5.9 Summary of the main results from the trial by Lao *et al.* (1999).

Outcome (after surgery)	Group A Acupuncture (n = 19) Mean (SE)	Group P Placebo (n = 20) Mean (SE)	Difference in means (A − P)	95% CI for the difference[†]	p-value
Length of time free from moderate pain*	172.9 (25.4)	93.8 (16.5)	79.1	18.2 to 140.0	0.01
Number of minutes before asking for pain relief	242.1 (23.5)	166.2 (17.2)	75.9	17.2 to 134.6	0.01
Number of pain medication tablets taken up to 24 hours after surgery[‡]	1.1	1.65	−0.55	−	0.05
Number of pain medication tablets taken 0–7 days after surgery	7.7 (2.0)	11.3 (3.0)	−3.6	−11.0 to 3.8	0.33

* It was stated that four patients given acupuncture never felt moderate pain compared to one patient in the placebo group.
† Confidence intervals were not given in the paper, but could be calculated from the reported results.
‡ It was not possible to calculate the 95% CI for the difference from results given in the paper.
SE: Standard error

difference is unlikely to be due to chance (p = 0.01). The true additional time before asking for pain relief could be as low as 17 minutes or as great as 135 minutes.

Pain medication used in the first 24 hours after surgery

On average, patients given acupuncture took about half a tablet less than those given placebo (−0.55) and this was statistically significant (p = 0.05). However a difference as small as this may not be considered clinically important.

Pain medication used in the 7 days after surgery

Patients given acupuncture took less pain medication in the 7 days after surgery; on average, they took about four fewer tablets. However, the difference was not statistically significant. This is reflected in the 95% confidence interval which indicates that the true effect could be that patients given acupuncture would take fewer tablets (up to 11) or that they would take more tablets (up to 4).

Number of patients experiencing moderate pain after surgery

Most patients experienced moderate pain. This was slightly less frequent in the acupuncture arm; 15 out of 19 (79%) in the acupuncture group and 19 out of 20 in the placebo group (95%), a difference of −16% with a confidence interval of −37% to +5%. The p-value for this comparison is 0.13, which is not statistically significant, so the observed difference could be a chance finding in this particular study. We are therefore unable to draw a firm conclusion on this aspect of pain. Either there really is no effect of acupuncture on moderate pain or there is a real difference, but the study was based on too few people to show this conclusively (see section on sample size).

Clinical importance and statistical significance

The differences between the groups in the time to experiencing pain, the time to asking for pain relief and the number of pain medication tablets taken within 24 hours were all statistically significant, whereas the amount of pain medication used in the 7 days following surgery and the number of patients free from moderate pain were not. The increase in length of time before pain became a problem was large. Patients given acupuncture were free from moderate pain for almost twice as long as patients given placebo; a difference of over 1 hour (172.9 versus 93.8 minutes). These effects could be considered clinically important. However, despite this delay in experiencing pain, there was little effect of treatment on overall consumption of pain medication or on the number of people who were pain free. This raises the question which of these is the most important clinical outcome in this study? This is discussed below in the section 'What does the study contribute to dental practice?'.

Side effects

The researchers reported that side effects (dizziness, heaviness, nausea and drowsiness) were only seen in the placebo group. The acupuncture group experienced more needle discomfort at the site of acupuncture, but this is expected. None of these side effects were quantified in the published paper.

How good is the evidence?

Box 5.10 summarises the main design and analysis considerations. For brevity, we have not expanded on them in the same way as in the previous section.

Sample size

Although the trial was relatively small (n = 39) it was still large enough to demonstrate statistically significant differences in some of the outcome measures. However, the small study size did produce results that had wide confidence intervals; for example, immediately after surgery the true extra pain-free time could be anywhere between 18 and 140 minutes. The comparison of the proportion of people who experienced moderate pain between acupuncture and placebo is not statistically significant (p-value = 0.13, not reported in the paper). Moderate pain was experienced by 16% fewer of the patients who received acupuncture than of those who did not. This is based on comparing 15/19 (79%) patients with 19/20 (95%), so it rests on a difference of only about 4 people. The confidence interval for the difference is wide (−37% to +5%) and implies that the sample is compatible with true values of the difference of anywhere

Box 5.10

Trial design	Was the study: randomised controlled blinded as far as possible	Yes Yes Yes, single-blind
Compliance	Was compliance similar between treatment arms? If not how might this affect the conclusions?	Yes
Lost to follow-up	Was follow-up similar between treatment arms? If not, how might this affect the conclusions?	There was no loss to follow-up
Sample size	Was the study large enough to detect a clinically important effect?	Yes for some (eg pain immediately after surgery) but not for others
Not for all the important outcomes Intention-to-treat analysis	Was the analysis on an intention-to-treat basis?	Yes

between up to 37% of patients in the acupuncture group having less pain or up to 5% having more pain. Although the confidence interval includes the no effect value, most of its range is in favour of acupuncture. In this situation we might want to follow this up by undertaking a larger study that would enable us to draw a firmer conclusion and provide a more precise estimate of the effect (i.e. narrower confidence intervals).

What does the study contribute to dental practice?

The results of the trial are likely to be reliable because patients were randomised and blind to treatment, thus avoiding the possible effects of bias. Acupuncture increased the time before feeling moderate pain and the time before requesting pain medication, and it slightly decreased the consumption of pain medication tablets in the first 24 hours. However, the evidence on whether it reduces the amount of pain medication used in the 7 days following surgery or the number of patients experiencing moderate pain is inconclusive. We could, therefore, deduce that it is the immediate effect on pain when the local anaesthetic is wearing off, that is of clinical relevance. Acupuncture may also reduce the amount of analgesics required at that time.

Who will the results apply to?

The patients in the trial were those who received surgery for an impacted third molar. The results may be applicable to all patients with this condition. They may also be applicable to other forms of oral surgery.

The trial was based on adults aged 18–40 years. Would the results be applicable to people aged 41–60 years? The generalisability of results from patients in one clinical trial to other patients deserves careful consideration before applying them to your practice.

Cost–benefit

The clinical benefits appear to outweigh any of the side effects. However, the end points of the amount of medication needed by seven days after surgery and the number of patients who remain pain-free could not be adequately addressed because the trial was too small. Further research could be done to investigate these more thoroughly.

Financial cost-effectiveness

The authors mention in the discussion that acupuncture is a cost-effective method of pain prevention. Although acupuncture could be considered an alternative to other forms of pain prevention or relief, its implementation would require an experienced acupuncturist to be present to deliver the treatment, and this would have a cost implication. Therefore, general dental surgeries may be unlikely to offer it.

Key points

- Clinical trials are the best way to determine the effectiveness of a new treatment or preventive regimen.
- Design elements central to clinical trials are:
  - randomisation (to produce trial arms with similar characteristics; avoids bias and confounding)
  - blinding (avoids bias)
  - control group (gives a standard for comparison)
  - clearly specified outcome measures
  - selection of patients (inclusion and exclusion criteria)
  - clearly specified intervention.
- Consider the size of the effect and 95% confidence interval (clinical importance).
- Consider whether the results could be chance findings (p-values).
- Statistical significance (p-value) is not the same as clinical importance (size of effect).
- Intention-to-treat analysis (maintains the balance achieved by randomisation; avoids bias).
- Sample size (was the trial large enough to detect a clinically important difference?).
- Could the results of the trial be applicable to your patients?

Appendix I is a table that could be completed when reading a clinical trial (using the study by Averley *et al.*). The table provide some guidelines on assessing such studies. If all the points cannot be completely addressed it does not necessarily mean that the conclusions are not valid or useful.

Acknowledgements

We are grateful to the journal *Archives of Otolaryngology—Head & Neck Surgery* and the publishers, the American Medical Association, for kindly giving permission to reproduce the abstract, methods section and Table 1 from the article by Lao *et al.* in this chapter.

Exercise

The following is a summary of a published randomised clinical trial.

Reference: Williams, B., Laxton, L., Holt, R.D. and Winter, G.B. Fissure sealants: a 4-year clinical trial comparing an experimental glass polyalkenoate cement with a bis glycidyl methacrylate resin used as fissure sealants. *Br Dent J* 1996;**180**:104–108.

What was the aim of the trial?
To compare the effect of two types of fissure sealants on developing caries in children.

What were the treatments?
The test sealant is an experimental glass polyalkenoate cement. The control sealant is a commonly used bis glycidyl methacrylate resin. The test sealant can be fixed under moist

Table 5.10   Summary of the main results on the fissure sealants (Williams *et al.*, 1996)*.

	Test sealant % (n) (a)	Control sealant % (n) (b)	Difference between the percentages (95% CI) (a − b)	p-value
Children seen 2 years later				
No. of teeth sealed	295	295		
Sealant lost	93 (274)	19 (55)	74 (69 to 80)	<0.0001
Caries/filled/extracted	7 (21)	2 (6)	5 (2 to 8)	0.003
Children seen 4 years later				
No. of teeth sealed	222	222		
Sealant lost	94 (208)	28 (62)	66 (59 to 72)	<0.0001
Caries/filled/extracted	10 (22)	7 (16)	3 (−2 to 8)	0.31
Children seen at both 2 and 4 years				
No. of teeth sealed	177	177		
Caries/filled/extracted:				
2 years later	6 (11)	1 (2)	5 (1 to 9)	0.01
4 years later	11 (20)	7 (12)	4 (−1 to 10)	0.14

*The number of children who attended for a dental examination was 157 (590 teeth) at 2 years and 117 (444 teeth) at 4 years; 93 children (354 teeth) attended both 2- and 4-year examinations.

conditions making it easier to apply than the standard sealant (control). Polyalkenoate contains fluoride and it has been suggested that the fluoride can be absorbed by the tooth.

How was the study conducted?
A total of 228 children aged 6–8 years from Suffolk, England. Each child received both the test and control sealants. Sealant was applied to the permanent molars. The test sealant was applied randomly to the the left or right side of the mouth and the control sealant applied to the opposite side (called a split or half mouth design). This meant that half the teeth were sealed with the test and half sealed with the control. All sealants were applied by two dentists responsible for the trial (authors of the paper).

What was the main outcome measure?
The main outcome measures were (i) the number of teeth which had lost the sealant and (ii) the number of teeth that had caries, were filled or had been extracted. Dental examinations were performed after 2 and 4 years in community dental clinics.

What are the main results?
Table 5.10 summarises the results on sealant retention and caries.

Questions

(1) Both the test and control sealants were given to each child (split mouth design). Why is this trial design better than one in which half the children had all their teeth sealed with the test sealant and half had all their teeth sealed with the control sealant (randomised two-arm design)?
(2) Comment on the proportion lost to follow-up (children who did not attend the 2- or 4-year examination).
(3) Interpret the results on sealent retention in Table 5.10.
(4) Interpret the results on caries in Table 5.10.
(5) What is the relative risk of losing sealants at 2 and at 4 years in the test sealant group compared to the control group?
(6) What is the relative risk of developing caries at 2 and at 4 years in the test sealant group compared to the control group?
(7) The following statements were reported in the paper:

> "A new glass ionomer material was compared with the standard bis GMA resin fissure sealant and after 2 and 4 years both were found to be equally effective at preventing caries."

> "Similar cariostasis was observed for the two materials at the end of 4 years despite marked differences in retention. Polyalkenoate cements probably should be regarded as fluoride depot materials rather than fissure sealants when used in this context."

Comment on these statements.

Answers on pp. 212–214

APPENDIX I. GUIDELINES FOR THE APPRAISAL OF A CLINICAL TRIAL USING THE TRIAL BY AVERLEY *ET AL.* (2004)

	Comments
1. Aim of the trial	
The aim is to treat patients with existing disease	Yes (anxiety over having dental treatment could be considered as existing disease). The aim is to reduce anxiety so that the dental treatment can be delivered successfully
Or the aim is to prevent disease from occurring	
2. Treatment	
How many treatment groups are there?	Three
What are the interventions?	Three gases: medical air, nitrous oxide (NO), nitrous oxide plus sevoflurane. Each was followed by intravenous midazolam
3. Randomisation	
(a) Were patients randomised to the treatment groups?	Yes
(b) Did randomisation produce groups with similar characteristics?	Yes, but there were two characteristics that appeared to differ (gender and baseline anxiety)
If not, do you think the differences are large enough to affect the results greatly?	No
4. Sample size	
(a) Is there a sufficient number of subjects?	Yes
(b) Have the authors described how large the trial needs to be?	Not in detail (but a pilot trial provided information on sample size)
5. Blinding	
Were the following blind to the treatment given to the patient?	
(a) The person giving the treatment	No
Patient	Yes
(b) The researcher making the assessment	Yes (the dentist)
(c) If any of the above were not blind, could they bias the results (need to consider how the outcome was measured)?	No. The anaesthetist could not be blind but he or she did not perform the surgery or take part in measuring the outcomes

(continued)

	Comments
6. Assessment of disease and treatments	
(a) What exactly is the disease of interest?	Anxiety
(b) Are diagnoses made or confirmed using standard criteria?	Yes
(c) Were a large number of patients lost to follow-up (i.e. it was not possible to record the main outcome)?	No
7. Results	
(a) Were the data analysed using an intention-to-treat analysis?	(b) No (but an intention-to-treat analysis gives similar results to those reported)
What is the size of the treatment effect?	Relative risk of 1.47 (nitrous oxide vs air); 1.73 (nitrous oxide plus sevoflurane vs air); 1.17 (nitrous oxide plus sevoflurane vs nitrous oxide)
(c) What is the 95% CI (the range of estimate of the true treatment effect)?	NO vs air 1.27 to 1.72 NO + sevo vs air 1.50 to 1.99 NO + sevo vs NO 1.09 to 1.25
(d) Are the results clinically important?	Yes
(e) Are the results likely to be due to chance?	No
(f) Are there any results on safety?	Yes
If so, what are the harmful effects of the treatment (consider size of the effect and if the results could be due to chance)?	Six cases of vomiting in the group that received nitrous oxide plus sevoflurane. An uncommon and short-term effect
8. The effect on dental practice	
(a) Are the study subjects similar to your population?	Likely to be the case
(b) If not, is there any reason why the results of the study would not be applicable to your population?	
(c) What are the implications of this and other studies on the management of your patients?	Nitrous oxide, with or without sevoflurane, is a safe and effective alternative to general anaesthesia for children who are anxious about receiving dental treatment

A randomised controlled trial of paediatric conscious sedation for dental treatment using intravenous midazolam combined with inhaled nitrous oxide or nitrous oxide/sevoflurane

P. A. Averley,[1] N. M. Girdler,[2] S. Bond,[3] N. Steen[4] and J. Steele[5]

1 Principle Dentist, Queensway Anxiety Management Clinic, 170 Queensway, Billingham UK
2 Consultant and Senior Lecturer, Sedation Department, School of Dental Science and Dental Hospital,
3 Professor and Head, School of Population and Health Sciences, 4 Centre for Health Service Research, 5 Professor of Health Service Research, School of Dental Science, University of Newcastle upon Tyne, UK

Summary

Failure of dental treatment due to anxiety is a common problem in children. The aim of this study was to establish whether the use of a combination of intravenous midazolam with inhalation agents (nitrous oxide alone or in combination with sevoflurane) was any more likely to result in successful completion of treatment than midazolam alone. A further aim was to evaluate the clinical viability of these techniques as an alternative to general anaesthesia. In total, 697 children too anxious for management with relative analgesia and requiring invasive dental procedure for which a general anaesthetic would usually be required, were recruited and randomly assigned to one of three groups given the following interventions: group 1 – a combination of inhaled medical air and titrated intravenous midazolam, group 2 – a combination of inhaled 40% nitrous oxide in oxygen and titrated intravenous midazolam, and group 3 – a combination of an inhaled mixture of sevoflurane 0.3% and nitrous oxide 40% in oxygen with titrated intravenous midazolam. The primary outcome measure was successful completion of the intended dental treatment with a co-operative child responsive to verbal commands. In group 1, 54%

(94/174 children) successfully completed treatment. In group 2, 80% (204/256 children) and in group 3, 93% (249/267 children) completed treatment. This difference was significant at the 1% level. Intravenous midazolam, especially in combination with inhaled nitrous oxide or sevoflurane and nitrous oxide, are effective techniques, with the combination of midazolam and sevoflurane the one most likely to result in successful treatment.

KEYWORDS *Anaesthesia, dental. Conscious sedation. Anaesthetics*: nitrous oxide, sevoflurane. *Benzodiazepines*: midazolam.

Correspondence to: Dr P. A. Averley
E-mail: patil@avcrley.cotn
Accepted: 14 March 2004

1 Child dental anxiety is widespread [1]. Many anxious children can be satisfactorily treated using behaviour management techniques combined with relative analgesia (RA), a simple technique using inhaled nitrous oxide and oxygen, but this approach is unsuccessful for some children [2]. In such cases, control of pain and anxiety poses a significant barrier to dental care and a dental general anaesthetic (DGA) is often seen as the only option. However, not only does DGA carry its own, well documented, risks but the dental treatment provided under DGA also tends to be more radical, with a greater proportion of extractions than fillings [3].

2 DGA has been successfully used when RA and behavioural management are ineffective [4], but the risks of DGA are significant. The UK Department of Health in its position document 'A Conscious Decision' recognised that although deaths were uncommon during and shorty after DGA (five deaths in dental practices in England in the 3 years 1996–1998), they were more likely than with any other method of pain and anxiety management [5]. Despite their infrequency, deaths associated with DGA have always been difficult to accept, and in many countries are now considered unacceptable, particularly when they occur in healthy children [6]. In the UK, DGA has been banned in non-hospital settings since 2002.

3 Two groups of children pose a particular management problem for dentists:

4 • Those who are extremely anxious and are unable to cope with treatment with behavioural management or RA.

• Those who require particularly invasive or extensive dental interventions.

If RA is ineffective and the risks of DGA unac- 4 ceptable, is there another option to manage the dental need of these individuals without admission to hospital?

In medical specialities, intravenous (i.v.) mida- 5 zolam is gaining popularity as a conscious sedation agent in children [7, 8]. The advantages of i.v. midazolam in children are the combination of rapid onset but short duration of action as well as haemodynamic stability. The safety and tolerability profile of midazolam in children has been described as 'comparable or superior to that observed in adults' [7].

By contrast, intravenous midazolam has not 6 been readily accepted as a means of conscious sedation for child dental patients, certainly in the UK and a number of other developed countries. The concerns are twofold. Firstly, it is argued that deeper levels of sedation than intended may be produced, and secondly, that the reaction of children to i.v. sedation may be unpredictable [9]. The evidence to support these concerns is limited and of low quality. Oral midazolam is, however, gaining popularity and is proving to be both safe and effective [10–12], but is not a realistic alternative to intravenous methods for the most anxious children. Given its successful use in other medical specialities [7, 8, 13], i.v. midazolam may be an important alternative, allowing conscious sedation for the child dental patient when DGA is considered the only other option.

Another possible solution to this clinical prob- 7 lem is the use of sevoflurane, a volatile anaesthetic agent with a sweet, non-pungent odour that can also be used for conscious sedation. It has a low blood-gas coefficient of 0.40 [14], allowing the depth of sevoflurane inhaled conscious sedation to be carefully controlled when used in subanaesthetic concentrations [15]. The sedative properties of inhaled sevoflurane have been investigated [15–19] whilst the use of inhaled sevoflurane in lower concentrations (0.1–0.3%) in addition to 40% nitrous oxide has been demonstrated to be successful as a paediatric conscious sedation technique with no adverse events [20, 21]. Like midazolam, sevoflurane may provide another option for conscious sedation in dentistry as an alternative to DGA.

8　Given the large variation in the needs of children, one conscious sedation technique is not enough to manage the needs of all anxious children. With the restriction in availability of DGA services in the UK and several other European countries, there is now an urgent need to develop and test a range of conscious sedation techniques for the large number of children who would otherwise require a DGA in a hospital setting. This study seeks to evaluate intravenous midazolam used in three different conscious sedation techniques. If effective and safe, these techniques have the potential to become part of the sedation armamentarium for a primary care setting, allowing the treatment of children who would otherwise require referral to a hospital for DGA.

9　The aim of this trial was to establish whether combinations of sedation agents, including intravenous midazolam, were any more likely to effect successful completion of treatment than midazolam alone when using conscious sedation techniques for the dental treatment of anxious children unsuitable for conventional behaviour management and RA techniques. A secondary aim was to assess the success of all of the techniques employed in the context of the only realistic alternative: a DGA in a hospital setting.

Materials and methods

10　This study tests the efficacy of three conscious sedation techniques. Completion of the planned dental treatment was the primary outcome measure. Secondary outcome measures were the poorest level of co-operation during treatment, the recovery time in minutes, the dose of midazolam used, the child's perceptions of anxiety and pain and the parent's satisfaction with the procedure.

11　The study was conducted in Queensway Anxiety Management Clinic (QAMC) in the North-East of England. This is part of a large primary care dental practice with a professional team of 10 dentists and six part time consultant anaesthetists who provide full time cover, 6 days a week. QAMC delivers dental care for more than 3000 children per year using a range of conscious sedation techniques. Appropriately trained and experienced dentists administer inhalation sedation with nitrous oxide or, if required for children over the age of 16 years, intravenous midazolam. For more anxious children who require complex techniques not suitable at present for general practice, operator sedation is not employed. These children are sedated in dedicated facilities with the addition of an appropriately trained and experienced consultant anaesthetist, an anaesthetist's assistant and a recovery nurse as part of the team [22].

12　Approval from the local research ethics committee and a licence from the medicines control agency were obtained prior to the start of the trial. Professionals involved in the study (dentists, anaesthetists, nurses and administrative staff) were formally trained in the study protocol and the use of its clinical scales before clinical work was undertaken. A pilot study to check procedures, refine criteria and to allow a power calculation for the main trial was undertaken [23].

Population and sample

13　Children were recruited aged between 6 and 14 years, who were referred by their general dental practitioner to QAMC for dental treatment using anxiety management. All children were assessed by one of 10 dentists experienced in the management of anxious children, and were entered into the trial if one or more of the following criteria were met (Fig. 1):

• The child's self-expressed level of anxiety scored four or more using the 10-point visual scale described by Wong & Baker [24].

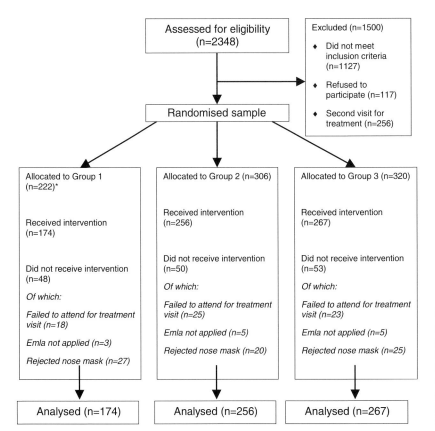

Figure 1 Flow diagram of the process through phases of the trial (enrolment, intervention allocation and data analysis). *Allocation to this group was stopped on the advice of the Data Monitoring Committee.

- The dentist's assessment of the child's co-operation scored three or more using the six-point co-operation behavioural scale described by Venham & Quatrocelli [25].
- The invasiveness of the planned dental procedure (for one visit) scored 10 or more using a numerical scale where one point is scored per quadrant of the mouth being treated, one point is scored per primary tooth treated, and two points are scored per permanent tooth treated.

14   Children were also required to have an adequate degree of comprehension and understanding regarding the treatment (if necessary with the support of interpretation services). They were also required to accept topical anaesthetic cream (EMLA®) applied to the dorsum of their hand prior to treatment and a nasal hood for the procedure. Any history of hypersensitivity to benzodi-azapines, sevoflurane, nitrous oxide or local anaesthetics (all are very rare) resulted in exclusion from the trial.

Verbal and written information about the study 15 was given to the parents of recruited children. Written informed consent/assent was obtained from recruited children/parents and EMLA® was supplied. Finally, a treatment appointment was arranged.

Randomisation and sedation technique

The children recruited were randomly allocated to 16 one of three groups using the Newcastle Centre for Health Services Research web based randomisation service. Randomisation was carried out by a nurse not connected with the study. A note of group allocation was placed in the patient record card in preparation for the appointment.

Journal paper

17　　Had there been no practical constraints, ran-domisation would have been carried out on the occasion of the visit for treatment after it had been ascertained that EMLA® cream had been applied, that the child would sit in the dental chair and accept the nose mask. For practical reasons, this was not possible and randomisation was carried out before the child's arrival for treatment. Children for whom treatment was not possible for the above reasons, or who failed to attend their treatment appointment, were not included in the analysis. The reason for withdrawal could not be influenced by the group allocation. For the pur-pose of the analysis, acceptance of the nose mask was regarded as the virtual point of randomisation and from that point on, all children were retained in the analysis on an 'intention to treat' basis.

18　　The three groups were:
- *Group 1*: Inhaled medical air at 6 l.min^{-1} for 2 min, followed by 0.5 mg of i.v. midazolam per minute, titrated to reach a clinical end point (Level 3 on the consciousness scale) [26].
- *Group 2*: Inhaled 40% nitrous oxide in oxygen at 6 l.min^{-1} for 2 min, followed by i.v. midazolam 0.5 mg.min^{-1}, titrated to reach a clinical end-point as described above.
- *Group 3*: Inhaled combination of 0.3% sevoflu-rane and 40% nitrous oxide in oxygen at 6 l.min^{-1} for 2 min, followed by midazolam 0.5 mg.min^{-1} titrated to reach a clinical endpoint as described above.

19　　EMLA® cream was applied to the dorsum of both hands of each child by a parent or guardian 1 h before treatment. At the start of the procedure, the child was asked to perform a baseline Eve's test (a simple test of spatial awareness in which the child touches the tip of his or her nose with a fore-finger with eyes closed) and then to breathe through a nasal mask. The anaesthetist then opened the envelope inside the record card identi-fying the technique randomly allocated and com-menced its administration for 2 min prior to can-nulation. Whilst all three groups received intra-venous midazolam, the positioning of the anaes-thetist and his/her equipment meant that the den-tist was blind to the gases being administered. Once the clinical endpoint was reached, a red car 20 toy was shown to the child for 5 s. The child was asked to recognise the object and memorise it for later in order to assess amnesia.

21　　Topical anaesthetic was then applied to the gum. Two minutes later the dentist injected lido-caine. During the procedure, the dentist main-tained verbal contact and ensured the child remained responsive to verbal commands. The dentist used calming suggestions and imagery to reassure the child and to distract him/her. At 5 min intervals, the treating dentist made a formal assessment of the child's co-operation using the six-point co-operation scale [25] and the child's level of consciousness using a six-point conscious-ness scale [26]. Children were maintained between level 3 (eyes open and responsive to verbal com-mands) and level 4 (eyes closed and responsive to verbal commands) on the consciousness scale. If necessary, the concentration of sevoflurane or nitrous oxide was reduced during the procedure if the child showed signs of over sedation (over level 3 on the consciousness scale) [26]. Throughout the procedure, the QAMC protocols of good seda-tion practice were employed [22].

22　　A Draeger Julian anaesthetic machine moni-tored pulse oximetry, automatic non-invasive blood pressure and ECG. The nasal hood was adapted to incorporate a probe to measure frac-tional inspired and end-tidal oxygen, carbon diox-ide, nitrous oxide, and sevoflurane. The anaes-thetist continuously monitored oxygen saturation, heart rate, ECG, capnography, fractional inspired sevoflurane and end-tidal sevoflurane and formally recorded them at 5 min intervals during treat-ment. Blood pressure was recorded once the clini-cal endpoint of sedation had been reached.

23　　If a child's level of co-operation rose to level 4 or greater ('reluctant' or worse) during treatment, the technique was deemed to have failed for the pur-poses of the study as at this point it becomes diffi-cult to provide effective dental care. The child then received appropriate anxiety management accord-ing to the QAMC protocols and the nature of the child's anxiety management subsequently employed was recorded. The intended dental treatment was carried out, limited only by the maximum dosage for local anaesthetic. If additional treatment was required, because of the extent of the treatment, a second visit was arranged but this visit was not included in the study.

24   After treatment, 100% oxygen was delivered through the nasal hood for 2 min before transfer on a trolley to the recovery room. The child was monitored during recovery by a nurse, who recorded a range of physiological and secondary outcome variables. The time taken to perform an Eve's test was recorded at 5-min intervals, as was the time taken to walk unaided across the recovery room, with close supervision. Before discharge, the child was asked to recall seeing the toy, to assess their level of amnesia. The child's level of anxiety and experience of pain was reassessed using the visual analogue scales previously reported [24]. Finally, the parent's opinion of the overall management of the child was recorded on a simple 5-point scale (1 = poor, through to 5 = excellent).

25   All data were recorded contemporaneously in ink on the anxiety management record sheet and the data stored in a locked cupboard prior to data entry.

Analytic strategy

26 An intention to treat analysis was performed. For each variable considered, initially all three groups were compared simultaneously to test the hypothesis that there were differences between the groups against the null hypothesis that there were no differences. For the key outcome measure (co-operation leading to successful completion of dental treatment) and for other binary variables, a Chi-squared test was undertaken. For continuous variables, a one-way analysis of variance with a standard F-test was undertaken. When the overall test indicated that the differences between groups were significant at the 5% level, groups were then compared pair-wise. For binary variables a 95% confidence interval for the relative risk (of success) between groups was calculated. For continuous variables, a 95% confidence interval for the difference in mean scores between the groups was calculated.

27   A fully independent Study Data Monitoring Committee, comprised of a statistician, a clinician and a lay member, was set up to monitor the progress of the trial. Their role was to ensure good practice by ensuring data quality during the trial and that the demographic breakdown of the groups supported random allocation. In addition, they monitored the outcome data and could advise the cessation of any arm of the trial on an ethical or statistical basis if the outcome was clearly less effective than those the other arms.

Results

28 The sample of 697 children was recruited over a 9-month period; their demographics, by test group, are shown in Table 1. Primary and secondary outcomes, by test group, are shown in Table 2. Children were generally healthy, 664 children were classed as American Society of Anaesthesiology (ASA) 1 and 33 children were ASA 11. The cases were well distributed in terms of age, assessment of co-operation and the invasiveness of the procedure undertaken, with no statistically significant differences between the three groups. There was an even distribution of dentists across the trial arms. There was a slight imbalance with respect to anxiety at assessment. Children were less anxious in Group 1, with a mean anxiety score of 5.6 (SD 2.0) than in Group 2 (6.1 (SD 1.7)) or Group 3 (6.0 (SD 1.9)). There was also an imbalance with respect to gender (see Table 1).

29   At the recommendation of the independent Study Data Monitoring Committee, an interim analysis of data was carried out by the committee and independent from the research team. It was decided by the committee that due to the high failure rate of Group 1, this arm of the study should be discontinued and the trial proceed with only Groups 2 and 3. As a result, the numbers of children recruited into Group 1 are lower than in Group 2 or 3.

30   Table 2 shows the results for both primary and secondary outcome measures. For the primary

Journal paper

Table 1 Baseline characteristics of the study groups.

Variable	Group 1: Air (n = 174)	Group 2: Nitrous oxide (n = 256)	Group 3: Sevoflurane (n = 267)	Overall test of difference between groups	Pair-wise comparison of groups 2 v 1	3 v 1	3 v 2
Sex (male); n (%)	81 (47%)	127 (50%)	103(39%)	$\chi^2_2 = 6.79$; p = 0.03	RR: 1 .07 (0.87, 1.30)	RR: 0.83 (0.67, 1.03)	RR; 0.78 (0.64, 0.95)
Age; mean (SD)	9.1 (2.7)	9.5 (2.7)	9.6 (2.5)	$F_{2,693} = 2.20$; p = 0.11			
Weight; mean (SD)	36.3 (13.4)	37.8 (14.1)	37.7 (14.0) (n = 251)	$F_{2,689} = 0.69$; p = 0.50			
Invasiveness of treatment; mean (SD)	8.9 (4.1)	9.7 (4.5) (n = 256)	9.8 (4.2) (n = 265)	$F_{2,692} = 2.65$; p = 0.07			
Anxiety at baseline assessment	5.6 (2.0)	6.1 (1.7)	6.0(1.9)	$F_{2,694} = 5.05$; p = 0.01	0.55 (0.21,0.90)	0.44 (0.07,0.80)	−0.16 (−0.42, 0.19)
Co-operation at baseline assessment	2.6(1.2)	2.8(1.1)	2.6 (1.2)	$F_{2,694} = 2.11$; p = 0.12			

measure of outcome, 54% (94/174 children) successfully completed treatment in Group 1, 80% (204/256 children) in Group 2 and 93% (249/267 children) in Group 3. The Chi-squared test indicated that differences between groups was significant at the 0.001% level. Given successful cannulation, the odds of successful treatment in Group 2 were not significantly greater than those in Group

1, with an odds ratio of 1.61 (95% CI: 0.96, 2.72). In this case, the p-value did not reach statistical significance (p = 0.075) and on the basis of the interval estimate of the odds ratio, we cannot exclude the possibility of a clinically important difference between the two treatment modes. Given successful cannulation, the odds of successful treatment in Group 3 were significantly

Table 2 Primary outcomes and secondary outcomes for successful cases.

	Group 1: Air (n = 174)	Group 2: Nitrous oxide (n = 256)	Group 3: Sevoflurane (n = 267)	Overall test of difference between groups	Pair-wise comparison of groups 2 v 1	3 v 1	3 v 2
Primary outcome							
Successful completion of treatment; n (%)	94 (54%)	204 (80%)	249 (93%)	$\chi^2_2 = 9.64$; p < 0.001	RR: 1.47 (1.27, 1.72)	RR:1.73 (1.50, 1.99)	RR: 1.17 (1.09, 1.25)
Secondary outcomes of successful cases							
Secondary outcomes of success	n = 94	n = 204	n = 249				
Total dose in mg of midazolam; mean (SD)	3.7(1.8)	3.2 (1.8)	2.6 (1.6)	$F_{2,544} = 16.1$; p < 0.001	−0.46 (−0.90, −0.03)	−1.08 (−1.47, −0.69)	−0.62 (−0.93, −0.31)
Poorest level of co-operation during treatment; mean (SD)	2.4 (0.7) (n = 93)	2.3 (0.8) (n = 203)	2.3 (0.7) (n = 248)	$F_{2,541} = 0.73$; p = 0.48			
Recovery time in min; mean (SD)	8.2 (5.6);	7.4 (3.5);	7.9 (4.2) (n = 247)	$F_{2,542} = 1 .36$; p = 0.26			
Child's perception of pain; mean (SD)	0.4 (1.1)	0.4(1.2)	0.4 (1.4)	$F_{2,544} = 0.05$; p = 0.95			
Anxiety reported by child; mean (SD)	0.8 (1.3)	0.8 (1.3)	0.8(1.3)	$F_{2,544} = 0.02$; p = 0.98			
Parent's satisfaction	4.7 (0.7)	4.8 (0.6)	4.8 (0.5)	$F_{2,544} = 0.70$; p = 0.50			
Any recall; n (%)	22 (24%) (n = 91)	27 (14%) (n= 194)	25 (10%) (n = 241)	$\chi^2_2 = 10.4$; p = 0.005	RR = 0.58 (0.35, 0.95)	RR = 0.43 (0.26, 0.72)	RR = 0.75 (0.45, 1.24)
Successful cannulation; n (%)	124(71%)	245 (95%)	262 (98%)	$\chi^2_2 = 101.4$; p = 0.001	RR = 1.34 (1.22, 1.48)	RR = 1.38 (1.25, 1.52)	RR = 1 .02 (0.99, 1.06)
Failed treatment after successful cannulation; n (%)	30 (24%) (n = 124)	41 (17%) (n = 245)	13(5%) (n = 262)	$\chi^2_2 = 31$; p = 0.001	RR = 0.69 (0.45, 1.95)	RR = 0.21 (0.11, 0.38)	RR = 0.30 (0.16, 0.54)

Table 3 Outcome techniques for failed treatments under initial sedation technique.

Variable	Group 1: I.v. midazolam & air(n = 174)	Group 2: I.v. midazolam & nitrous oxide (n = 256)	Group 3: I.v. midazolam & nitrous oxide & sevoflurane (n = 267)
Addition of sevoflurane and nitrous oxide allowing completion of treatment	59	24	n/a
Addition of other i.v. agent (maintaining consciousness level 4) allowing completion of treatment	10	13	11
Referral back to own dentist	6	8	4
Referral for General anaesthetic	5	7	4
Total number of failures	80	52	19

greater than those in Group 1, with an odds ratio of 6.33 (95% CI: 3.18, 12.65). Given successful cannulation, the odds of successful treatment in Group 3 were significantly greater than those in Group 2, with an odds ratio of 3.94 (95% CI: 2.06, 7.52).

Of the 151 failed treatments shown in Table 3, 59 children in Group 1 and 24 children in Group 2 were successfully treated with the addition of sevoflurane and nitrous oxide in oxygen. A further 34 children (including Group 3 failures) were managed with an alternative conscious sedation technique (by administration of additional sedation agents), ensuring at all times that consciousness did not drop below level 4 on the consciousness scale [26]. Eighteen children who could not be managed using conscious sedation techniques were referred back to their own general dental practitioner as they did not meet the clinic referral protocol for a DGA because there was no need for urgent treatment. Sixteen children required referral to a hospital setting for DGA.

The analysis of secondary outcomes is restricted to subjects who underwent a successful procedure (Table 2). There were significant differences between groups (p < 0.001) in the amount of midazolam required. The dose of midazolam was not weight determined but titrated to a clinical endpoint, and the pair-wise comparisons indicate children who received sevoflurane (Group 3) needed less midazolam then children in the other two groups. There was no difference (p = 0.48) between the Groups for the poorest level of co-operation recorded amongst those who were treated successfully. Differences in recovery times were not statistically significant (p = 0.26). There was no statistical significance in child perception of pain (p = 0.95) and anxiety in recovery (p = 0.98) or parent's satisfaction (p = 0.5).

All children were responsive to verbal commands throughout the duration of the procedure and during recovery (no children scored greater than 4 on the consciousness scale). No significant adverse events were encountered during the study. One child in Group 1 suffered a vaso-vagal attack during cannulation, and six children in Group 3 vomited clear fluids after treatment. All children remained well saturated and within acceptable limits for conscious sedation during treatment and in recovery. In total, 98% of children had an oxygen saturation of 98% or above. The lowest saturation of 94% was recorded in one child in Group 1. Heart rates and blood pressure remained ± 20% of normal base values throughout treatment and recovery for every patient.

Children in all groups exhibited good amnesia as would be expected with the use of midazolam. However, 30/124 children (24%) in Group 1, 27/194 children (14%) in Group 2 and 25/241 children (10%) in Group 3 had some recall of the dental procedure. This difference was significant between the groups (p = 0.005).

35   There were significant differences between groups (p < 0.001) when the level of co-operation during cannulation was compared. In Group 1, 71% (124/174) co-operated to allow successful cannulation compared with 95% (245/256) in Group 2 and 98% (262/267) in Group 3.

Discussion

36 The findings from this single centre randomised control trial clearly show that inhalation support provided by a combination of inhalation sedation and intravenous midazolam rather than intravenous midazolam alone, improves co-operation during cannulation, improves the level of co-operation during the dental procedure, resulting in a higher rate of successfully completed treatment, reduces the dose of midazolam required and produces good amnesia. Delivered in a primary care setting with involvement of anaesthetists, these techniques are effective and apparently safe. The clinical significance of this is that it potentially reduces the need for hospital referral for a DGA.

37   Adverse events are rare in dental anaesthesia, and a definitive evaluation of safety requires a long history of treatment using a given technique. Whilst a trial of this size cannot assess the frequency of possible adverse events, the results presented here indicate a safe technique. The conscious sedation techniques practised ensured co-operation and consciousness throughout the procedure and full control of protective reflexes. This is in stark contrast to DGA, and also in contrast to the practice of 'deep sedation'.

38   Only minor adverse events were recorded, and the only ones that had clinical relevance were six cases where children vomited clear fluids, all of which occurred in the midazolam/nitrous oxide/sevoflurane group. While the numbers are too small for comparative analysis, they suggest that there may be a greater risk of vomiting where these agents are used in combination. This occurred in just over 2% of such cases so the overall prevalence is very low. Nevertheless, where

more than one agent is used we would recommend that the patient is starved before the procedure as a precautionary measure in accord with the protocol used in this study.

39   It is widely accepted that conscious sedation is safer than general anaesthetic [2, 23, 26–30], However, poorly controlled conscious sedation may result in 'deep sedation' or even general anaesthesia with all its attendant risks [2, 31]. The sedationist must be able to exert a fine control over the level of sedation and the margin of safety between sedation and anaesthesia must be wide enough to prevent unintended loss of consciousness occurring. Such techniques are not particularly difficult and can be appropriate for a primary care setting, but do need to be practised by trained personnel. Children requiring more complex techniques for effective sedation, involving combinations of drugs such as those used in this trial, should be treated in specialist centres with appropriately trained and experienced teams where a trained anaesthetist is present. However, treatment does not need to be undertaken in a hospital setting and does not require admission.

40   The evidence from this trial suggests that, provided proper care and attention are exercised, intravenous sedation in combination with inhaled agents may be a useful alternative to DGA. The results of this trial adds to the evidence base for sedation techniques which can be used to help children who fail to accept dental treatment using local anaesthetic alone or supplemented with conventional relative analgesia sedation. The development of guidelines on paediatric conscious sedation needs to be an ongoing process based on new evidence such as that presented in this paper [2, 32].

Acknowledgements

We thank all the patients involved in this study. We are grateful for the support of an NHS R & D National Primary Care Researcher Developers Award (2002). Thanks to dental surgeons: Dr M. Hanlon, Dr I. Lane, Dr R. Hobman, Dr U. Mansoor, Dr B. Smith, Dr J. Sykes and A. Weston for their valuable contribution. In addition to consultant anaesthetists Dr S. Gooneratne, Dr G. Lahoud, Dr H. Mohan and Dr I. Riddle for their support and advice. We thank all the staff at QAMC for their hard work and Abbott Laboratories for providing the sevoflurane.

References

1 Veerkamp JS, Gruythuysen RJ, van Amerongen WE, *et al.* Dental treatment of fearful children using nitrous oxide. Part 2: The parent's point of view, *Journal of Dentistry for Children* 1992; **59**: 115–9.

2 Scottish Intercollegiate Guidelines Network. *Safe Sedation of Children Undergoing Diagnostic and Therapeutic Procedures. A National Clinical Guideline.* NHS Scotland, Edinburgh, 2002.

3 Harrison M, Nutting L. Repeat general anaesthesia for paediatric dentistry. *British Dental Journal* 2000; **189**; 37–9.

4 Holt RD, Chidiac RH, Rule DC. Dental treatment for children under general anaesthesia in day care facilities at a London dental hospital. *British Dental Journal* 1991; **170**: 262–6.

5 Department of Health. *A Conscious Decision. A Review of the Use of General Anaesthesia and Sedation in Primary Dental Care.* London: Department of Health, 2000.

6 Worthington LM, Flynn PJ, Strunin L. Death in the dental chair: an avoidable catastrophe? *Anaesthesia* 1998; **80**: 131–2.

7 Rosen DA, Rosen KR. Intravenous conscious sedation with midazolam in paediatric patients. *International Journal of Clinical Practice* 1998; **52**: 46–50.

8 Shannon M, Albers G, Burkhart K, *et al.* Safety and efficacy of flumazenil in the reversal of benzodiazepine-induced conscious sedation. The Flumazenil Pediatric Study Group. *Journal of Paediatrics* 1997; **131**: 582-6.

9 Hosey MT. UK National Clinical Guidelines in Paediatric Dentistry. *International Journal of Paediatric Dentistry* 2002; **12**: 359–72.

10 Erlandsson AL, Backman B, Stenstrom A, *et al.* Conscious sedation by oral administration of midazolam in paediatric dental treatment. *Swedish Dental Journal* 2001; **25**: 97–104.

11 Wilson KE. Welbury RR, Girdler NM. A randomised, controlled, crossover trial of oral midazolam and nitrous oxide for paediatric dental sedation. *Anaesthesia* 2002; **57**:860–7.

12 Wilson KE, Welbury RR, Girdler NM. A study of the effectiveness of oral midazolam sedation for orthodontic extraction of permanent teeth in children: a prospective, randomised, controlled, crossover trial. *British Dental Journal* 2002; **192**: 457–62.

13 Alcaino EA. Conscious sedation in paediatric dentistry: current philosophies and techniques. *Australia College of Dental Surgery* 2000; **15**: 206–10.

14 Rang HP, Dale MM, Ritter JH. *Pharmacology*, 4th edn. London: Churchill Livingstone, 2001.

15 Haraguchi N, Furusawa H, Takezaki R, *et al.* Inhalation sedation with sevoflurane: a comparative study with nitrous oxide. *Journal of Oral Maxillofacial Surgery* 1995; **53**: 24–6.

16 Ganzberg S, Weaver J, Beck FM, McCaffrey G. Use of sevoflurane inhalation sedation for outpatient third molar surgery. *Anaesthesia* 1999; **46**: 21–9.

17 Hoerauf KH, Hartmann T, Zavrski A, *et al.* Occupational exposure to sevoflurane during sedation of adult patients. *International Journal of Occupational Environmental Health* 1999; **72**: 174–7.

18 Ibrahim AE, Taraday JK, Kharasch ED. Bispectral index monitoring during sedation with sevoflurane, midazolam, and propofol. *Ancsthcsiology* 2001; **95**: 1151–9.

19 Katoli T, Bito H, Sato S. Influence of age on hypnotic requirement, bispectral index, and 95% spectral edge frequency associated with sedation induced by sevoflurane. *Anesthesiology* 2000; **92**: 55–61.

20 Lahoud GY, Averley PA, Hanlon MR. Sevoflurane inhalation conscious sedation for children having dental treatment. *Anaesthesia* 2001; **56**: 476–80.

21 Lahoud GY, Averley PA. Comparison of sevoflurane and nitrous oxide mixture with nitrous oxide alone for inhalation conscious sedation in children having dental treatment: a randomised controlled trial. *Anaesthesia* 2002; **57**: 446–50.

22 Averley PA. Queensway Anxiety Management Clinic Referral Protocols, 2003. *http://www.anxietymanagement.co.uk*

23 Averley PA, Lane I, Sykes J. A RCT pilot study to test the effects of intravenous midazolam as a conscious sedation technique for anxious children requiring dental treatment; An alternative to general anaesthesia. *British Dental Journal* 2004; NHS Scotland, Edinburgh.

24 Wong DL, Baker CM. Children's visual and verbal rating scale. *Paediatric Nursing* 1988; **14**: 1.

Journal paper

25 Venham L, Quatrocelli S. The young child's response to repeated dental procedures. *Journal of Dental Research* 1977; **56**: 734–8.

26 Girdler NM, Hill CM. *Sedation in Dentistry,* 1st edn. London: Wright publications, 1998.

27 American Academy of Paediatric Dentistry. *Clinical Guideline on the Elective Use of Conscious Sedation, Deep Sedation and General Anaesthesia in Paediatric Dental Patients.* AAPD, Chicago, USA, 1998.

28 Department of Health Review Group. *A Conscious Decision.* London: Department of Health UK, 2000.

29 Department of Health. Department of Health circular (from the director of Health Services), 2001; letter to all GDP's, Health Authorities, NHS trusts and Dental Practice Board. London: Department of Health, 2001.

30 Malamed SF. *Sedation. A Guide to Patient Management,* 3rd edn. Mosby, Boston, USA, 1995.

31 Morton NS, Oomen GJ. Development of a selection and monitoring protocol for safe sedation of children. *Paediatric Anaesthesia* 1998; **8**: 65–8.

32 General Dental Council. Maintaining Standards November, 2001. London: General Dental Council. 2001.

Evaluation of Acupuncture for Pain Control After Oral Surgery

A Placebo-Controlled Trial

Lixing Lao, PhD, LAc; Stewart Bergman, DDS; Gayle R. Hamilton, PhD;
Patricia Langenberg, PhD; Brian Sermon, MD

Background: Acupuncture is increasingly being used by the general population and investigated by conventional medicine; however, studies of its effects on pain still lack adequate control procedures.

Objectives: To evaluate the (1) efficacy of Chinese acupuncture in treating postoperative oral surgery pain, (2) validity of a placebo-controlled procedure, and (3) effects of psychological factors on outcomes.

Design: Randomized, double-blind, placebo-controlled trial.

Setting: Dental School Outpatient Clinic, University of Maryland at Baltimore.

Participants: Thirty-nine healthy subjects, aged 18 to 40 years, assigned to treatment (n = 19) and control (n = 20) groups.

Main Outcome Measures: Patients' self-reports of time until moderate pain, time until medication use, total pain relief, pain half gone, and total pain medication consumption.

Results: Mean pain-free postoperative time was significantly longer in the acupuncture group (172.9 minutes) than in the placebo group (93.8 minutes) (*P* = .01), as was time until moderate pain (*P* = .008). Mean number of minutes before requesting pain rescue medication was significantly longer in the treatment group (242.1 minutes) than in the placebo group (166.2 minutes) (*P* = .01), as was time until medication use (*P* = .01). Average pain medication consumption was significantly less in the treatment group (1.1 tablets) than in the placebo group (1,65 tablets) (*P* = .05). There were no significant berween-groups differences on total-pain-relief scores or pain-half-gone scores (*P* > .05). Nearly half or more of all patients were uncertain of or incorrect about their group assignment. Outcomes were not associated with psychological factors in multivariate models.

Conclusions: Acupuncture is superior to the placebo in preventing postoperative dental pain; no-insertion placebo procedure is valid as a control.

Arch Otolaryngol Head Neck Surg. 1999,125:567-572

PATIENTS AND METHODS

Procedures

Detailed methods and materials are described in our previous report.[23] In brief, all patients were recruited from the out-patient pool of the Oral and Maxillofacial Surgery Clinic at the University of Maryland at Baltimore Dental School Patients were aged 18 to 40 years, in good health

(American Society of Anesthesiologists class I or II), eligible for extraction of 1 mandibular (lower) partial bony impacted third molar, and had no history of prior treatment with acupuncture. Excluded patients were those who presented with any oral dental disease, those taking medications that might confound the results, those with a history of bleeding diathesis or allergy to the medication used in the study, or women who were pregnant or lactating. No race or sex was excluded from the study. After initial screening, the purposes and procedures of the study were explained, and the patients read, understood, and signed an informed consent that was approved by the Institutional Review Board of the University of Maryland. The dental procedure was performed by one surgeon (S.B.) blinded to treatment assignment. All patients were given the same local anesthetic of 3% mepivacaine hydrochloride (Carbocaine) without any vasoconstrictor. No other preoperative medication was used.

2   The patients were randomly assigned to either real acupuncture or placebo acupuncture immediately after the surgical removal of a partial bony impacted third molar. Randomized blocks of 4 and 6 were used to attain balanced allocation. Patients were assigned to a treatment group using sequentially numbered opaque sealed envelopes. A licensed acupuncturist (L.L.) administered all treatments and was the only investigator who knew what type of treatment the patient received. In the real acupuncture group, the acupuncture points *Hegu* (LI 4), *Jiache* (St 6), *Xiaguan* (St 7), and *Yifeng* (SJ 17) were used unilaterally on the tooth extraction side. All needles remained in place for 20 minutes, and each was manually manipulated (no electrical stimulation was applied) for 20 to 30 seconds 3 times: immediately after insertion, at the midpoint, and at the end of treatment. The "de qi" sensation (a sensation of soreness, numbness, or distention at the needling site) was obtained for each manipulation. In the placebo group, the procedure was identical to that used in the treatment group except without needle insertion into the skin. An empty plastic needle

tube was tapped on the bony area next to each acupuncture point to produce some discernible sensation, and a needle with a piece of adhesive tape was then taped to the derma surface for 20 minutes. Manipulations were made by palpating the surface of the skin with a blunt dental instrument at the same 3 points in time as the treatment group. In both groups, the patients' eyes were covered with patches so they could not view the treatment procedure. A pair of electrodes from a mock electrical stimulator was attached to the ends of the needles in the real and placebo acupuncture groups. A second treatment was given after patients reported moderate pain on a 4-point scale. For each subject, the second treatment was the same as the first treatment (acupuncture or placebo).

ASSESSMENTS AND FOLLOW-UP

Pain

The pain model used[29,30] was developed by 3 Cooper and Beaver and is widely accepted by both the pharmaceutical Industry and the Food and Drug Administration to assess oral pain medication. Pain intensity was evaluated on a 4-point scale (0 indicates none; 1, slight/mild; 2, moderate; 3, severe) using a standardized questionnaire administered by a blinded clinical assistant.[19,30] Pain assessments were in 2 steps: (1) every 15 minutes after the first treatment until the reported pain reached a moderate level, at which time the patient had a second treatment, and (2) every 15 minutes for 3 hours after the second treatment. If a patient indicated no pain relief 30 minutes after the treatment, or if the intensity of pain increased, a standard analgesic medication (acetaminophen, 600 mg, with codeine, 60 mg) was administered at the patient's request. In this situation, pain scores following rescue medication were carried through as moderate or severe, according to the patient report at the time of the rescue medication request.[30] For each patient, assessments included self-reports of time until moderate pain, time until medication use, total pain medication consumption, total pain relief, and pain half gone.

4 Patients were observed on-site for 3 hours after the second acupuncture treatment or 6 hours after the first treatment if the pain did not reach a moderate level. They were asked to continue recording their pain levels every hour for 24 hours after treatment and to provide global assessments daily for 7 days. Patients who fell asleep and did not complete the evaluation form were assigned a rating of pain intensity equal to the last recording before falling asleep.[30] The follow-up forms were turned in on the seventh day when the patient returned to the clinic for suture removal.

Determining risk factors for and causes of disease

Clinical trials provide a powerful tool for evaluating treatments because they are **experimental** studies which allow us to assign interventions to people. Randomisation is used to make sure that the groups of people compared are likely to be similar in all characteristics except the treatment. Identifying causes of disease is more complex than investigating treatments because we cannot perform experiments that expose people to potential harm.

The causal links between smoking and disease were not accepted for many decades – if experiments had been possible the link would have been easier to establish. For example, the simplest way to determine if smoking causes periodontitis would be to select a group of adults without periodontitis, randomise half to smoke cigarettes and the other half not to, and then follow them for, say, 5 years. We would then compare smokers and non-smokers and see how many developed periodontitis in each group. Of course, this experiment is not possible because making people smoke cigarettes would be unethical. When investigating causes of a disease we must therefore rely on **observational** studies, where we observe, for example smokers and non-smokers, and see who gets the disease.

The main disadvantage of observational studies in contrast to experimental studies is that we cannot minimise differences in characteristics in the comparison groups by using randomisation, so there will be other factors besides the exposure of interest that may be influencing the results. When investigating the effect of smoking on periodontitis and smoking, we cannot randomise people to smoking or non-smoking in our observational study, so there will be many differences in characteristics between smokers and non-smokers. This makes it harder to establish that any difference between the groups in the level of periodontitis is actually caused by smoking and not by some other factor. For example, we could find that smokers are older than non-smokers and that periodontitis levels are generally higher in older people. Even if the smoking group have more periodontitis, how can we tell whether this is really due to smoking or simply because the smoking group is older?

When we investigate the causes of a disease we are usually interested in its relationship with a specified **exposure**, for example smoking, fluoride or diet. There may be many different exposures that affect the risk of having a disease. When some other factor is distorting the relationship between the exposure and the outcome, this is called **confounding**. A confounding factor can either obscure the relationship of interest or spuriously create one. It is something that is inherent to most observational studies and difficult, or impossible, to avoid. Randomised trials are rarely affected by confounding because the process of randomising usually removes this effect.

The purpose of this chapter is to introduce the two main types of observational study that are used to help determine causes of disease – **cohort** and **case–control** studies. In dental research, cohort studies are more common than case–control studies, therefore this chapter will be based around one full paper from a cohort study and on parts of another paper from a case–control study. Before these are discussed we will distinguish between association and causality, and describe confounding and how it can adversely affect results.

ASSOCIATION, CAUSALITY AND CONFOUNDING

Association and causality

Many research studies report findings on the risk of oral disease and exposure to a specified factor. The results of a study may show that there is an **association** between the exposure and the disease; more of the people who are exposed have the disease. We cannot automatically assume from this that the exposure causes the disease. When we talk about an exposure **causing** a certain disease, what do we really mean? A **cause** implies that there is an underlying biological mechanism between the exposure and the disease. Thus, if the exposure is removed the risk of the disease will reduce. **Association** simply describes a relationship between a factor and disease but it does not necessarily indicate the presence of a biological pathway. If a factor and disease are associated with each other there may or may not be a causal relationship. We illustrate this with the example below.

Example: use of sunscreen and the risk of drowning

As the months proceed toward summer, sales of sunscreen increase. Death from drowning also increases noticeably in the same time period. This is a real relation (it is not due to chance) so can we say that using sunscreen **causes** people to drown? The answer is NO. Although use of sunscreen is **associated** with drowning, there is no reason why it would lead directly to drowning. The association arises through association with a third factor, the weather. Warm weather causes people to use sunscreen; warm weather also makes people want to swim. So there is a direct link between warm weather and each of the factors. There is no direct link between using sunscreen and drowning. If sunscreen were banned the number of people who drown would not necessarily decrease. So there is an *association* between sunscreen and drowning, but it is not causal, it is entirely due to the *confounding* effect of warm weather.

Confounding

Confounding arises when the exposure and the outcome are *both* related to some other factor (consumption of sunscreen and drowning are both related to warm weather). As we saw above, confounding can sometimes explain all of an association between

Table 6.1 Hypothetical study to illustrate the death rate in smokers and non-smokers according to drinking status.

	Non-smokers			Smokers			Relative risk* (B ÷ A)
	No. of men	No. of deaths	Death rate per year (A)	No. of men	No. of deaths	Death rate per year (B)	
All	1000	7	7 per 1000	1000	14	14 per 1000	2
Non-drinkers	660	0	0 per 1000	340	0	0 per 1000	Not defined†
Drinkers	340	7	21 per 1000	660	14	21 per 1000	1

* The ratio of the death rate in smokers compared to the rate in non-smokers.
† Not defined because it involves dividing zero by zero.

an exposure and an outcome. More often, part of the association is explained by a confounder. For example, periodontal disease in pregnant women is associated with preterm low birth-weight in infants. However, smoking is also associated with preterm low birth-weight and with periodontal disease, so part of the association between periodontal disease and low birth-weight could be due to smoking. The following two examples illustrate how confounding works.

Example: smoking and cirrhosis of the liver

Observational studies show the death rate from cirrhosis of the liver to be greater in smokers than that in non-smokers, and this provides evidence for an association. Table 6.1 shows hypothetical data of 1000 male non-smokers and 1000 male smokers. The relative risk of cirrhosis is 2 in smokers compared with non-smokers. However, there is another factor, alcohol consumption, that should be taken into account. Alcohol consumption is a potential confounding factor in the association between cirrhosis and smoking because:

- smokers are more likely to drink alcohol than non-smokers
- people who drink alcohol are more likely to get cirrhosis than non-drinkers.

Therefore, the observed association between smoking and death from cirrhosis could be due to drinking. To check this, we examine the relation between smoking and cirrhosis in drinkers and non-drinkers *separately* – this is called **stratification**. Table 6.1 shows the death rates for cirrhosis stratified by drinking status. The death rate for drinkers and non-drinkers combined is 7 per 1000 in non-smokers and 14 per 1000, twice as high, among smokers. When the death rates are stratified by drinking, there is no association between smoking and cirrhosis. Looking at non-drinkers only, the death rate is the same in non-smokers and smokers (0 per 1000). Looking at drinkers only, the death rate is also the same in non-smokers and smokers (21 per 1000). In this way we can say that we have examined the effect of smoking on cirrhosis after **allowing** (or **adjusting**) for drinking. If we had not allowed for drinking as a confounder we would have concluded, incorrectly, that smoking causes cirrhosis.

Table 6.2 Results on periodontitis, smoking and occupation from the study by Sheiham (1971).

(i) Periodontitis and smoking

	Smokers (n = 247)	Non smokers (n = 248)	
Mean periodontal index	4.33	3.56	Difference +0.77 (p-value <0.01)

Smokers have a significantly higher periodontal index than non-smokers

(ii) Occupation and smoking

Occupation	Smokers	Nonsmokers	Percentage of workers who smoke
Manual	167	149	53%
Non-manual	80	99	45%
			Relative risk 1.18 (p = 0.08)

Manual workers are more likely to smoke

(iii) Occupation and periodontitis

	Manual	Non-manual	
Mean periodontal index	4.18	3.55	Difference +0.63

Manual workers have a higher periodontal index

(iv) Periodontitis and smoking, allowing for occupation

	Mean periodontal index		
	Smokers	Nonsmokers	Difference
Manual	4.44	3.88	+0.56
Non-manual	4.11	3.09	+1.02

When manual workers and non-manual workers are looked at separately, smokers have a higher periodontal index than non-smokers

Example: periodontitis and cigarette smoking

An example of confounding from the dental literature is presented in a cross-sectional study that examined the association between periodontitis and cigarette smoking in a group of 495 workers, in Northern Ireland (Sheiham A. Periodontal disease and oral cleanliness in tobacco smokers. *Br Dent J* 1971;**42**:259–263). Periodontitis was quantified by a 'periodontal index'; the higher the index the greater the severity of the disease. Table 6.2 shows results that were derived from the paper. The main result showed that the mean periodontal index is greater in smokers (4.33) than in non-smokers (3.56) and that the difference is statistically significant – evidence for an association between periodontitis and smoking.

However, there was another factor, occupation, which could have acted as a confounder because it was associated with both smoking and periodontitis:

- Manual workers were more likely to be smokers than non-manual workers (smoking prevalence 53% in manual workers versus 45% in non-manual workers, a relative risk of 1.18).

- Manual workers tended to have more severe periodontitis than non-manual workers (mean periodontal index 4.18 versus 3.55, respectively, a difference of 0.63).

   To investigate the effect of confounding the data were **stratified** by presenting the results on periodontitis and smoking separately for each occupational group. The mean difference in periodontal index between smokers and non-smokers was +0.56 in manual workers and +1.02 in non-manual workers. The periodontal index remains higher in smokers than in non-smokers in each group of workers. Therefore, the conclusion that periodontitis is associated with smoking is maintained after allowing for occupation.
   A factor can only be a confounder if it is associated with both the exposure of interest and the disease. Of course, we can only allow for confounding factors if we know of them. It is therefore possible that a study may show an association and although we have allowed for some confounders, there may be others of which we are unaware.

COHORT STUDIES

What is a cohort study?

We saw that in a clinical trial we intervene and provide a treatment. In a cohort study there is no intervention, we just observe what is happening. A cohort study is said to be **observational** whereas a clinical trial is **interventional**. In a cohort study, people are disease-free at the start of the study and we are interested in finding out the number of *new* cases of disease (**incidence**) that develop over the course of the study. We then see whether the incidence differs between people who were or were not exposed to the factor of interest during the course of the study. Figure 6.1 shows the main features of a typical cohort study.

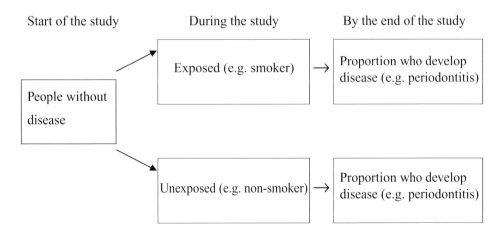

Figure 6.1   Illustration of the design of a cohort study.

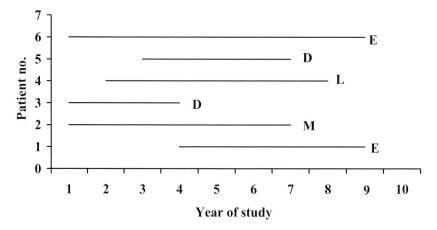

Figure 6.2 Illustration of how people can leave and enter a cohort study (six subjects). See text for explanation of abbreviations.

What is meant by 'follow-up time'?

At the start of any cohort study information is obtained on each person about the exposure of interest (for example smoking status). They are also examined or questioned to ensure that they do not have the disease of interest. They are then **followed up**, usually for several months or years, and during this time a record is kept both of their exposure and whether they develop the disease. Often, in studies with a long period of follow-up, individuals are followed for different lengths of time. Individuals may be recruited over a fixed period of time (not everyone enters the study at the same point in time), then followed up until the date when the study ends. Figure 6.2 illustrates how individuals can enter and leave a cohort study. Follow-up time starts when the subject enters the study and ends when any of the following occur:

- the study ends (E)
- the subject cannot be contacted to ascertain their state of health (they are said to be 'lost to follow-up') (L)
- they are diagnosed with the disease of interest (D)
- they have died (M).

The time a person spends in the study during which they are at risk is called the **period at risk**. Each year that an individual is at risk is called a **person-year-at-risk**. In the simplest case, if 10 people are each followed for exactly five years (or 25 people for 2 years), there are 50 person-years. However, it is rare that everyone has been in the study for the same length of time; person-years-at-risk take into account both the number of people and how long each has been in the study. It reflects the fact that someone who participated for 15 years would provide more information than someone who only participated for 3 years.

Rates of disease

The **rate** of occurrence of an outcome event is the number of *new* events occurring during a *specified period of time*. For example, in the UK in 2001[1] there were 2868 newly diagnosed cases of oral cancer among 28 579 869 males[1]; the **incidence rate** is thus 10.0 per 100 000 men per year [(2868 ÷ 28 579 869) × 100 000]. The number of new cases in females was 1532 among 30 209 325 individuals, an incidence rate of 5.1 per 100 000 females per year[1]. Rates are also used to describe the number of deaths due to a particular disease. The number of deaths from oral cancer among all males in the UK in 2003 was 1018, so the **mortality rate** is 3.5 per 100 000 males per year.

In Chapter 2, we saw how to calculate a relative risk from two proportions. We can do the same thing using two rates. To calculate the relative risk of oral cancer incidence in men compared with women we take the ratio of the two rates.

$$\text{Relative risk} = \frac{\text{Rate in men}}{\text{Rate in women}} = \frac{10.0}{5.1} = 2.0$$

Men were about twice as likely to develop oral cancer as women in 2001.

AN EXAMPLE OF A COHORT STUDY

Please read the paper (reproduced on pp. 144–151) before proceeding.

> Reference: Pitiphat, W., Merchant, A.T., Rimm, E.B. and Joshipura, K.J. Alcohol consumption increases periodontitis risk. *J Dent Res* 2003;**82**:509–513.

What is the aim of the study?

The authors state that their aim was to examine the association between alcohol use and the risk of periodontitis (*paragraph 1*). Although the study is based on male health professionals we are really interested in the effect of alcohol use on periodontitis in all adults.

How was the study conducted?

This is a **cohort study** (sometimes called a longitudinal or prospective study) based on 51 529 male health professionals in the USA aged 40–75 years in 1986. Of these, 39 461 were included in the present study (*paragraph 3*). The cohort included dentists, veterinarians, pharmacists, optometrists, osteopathic physicians and podiatrists (*paragraph 2*). Cohort studies are often based on specific groups of workers who belong to professional organisations, because these people tend to continue to have contact with their professional body and are therefore easier to follow up over long periods of time. This cohort has been followed since 1986.

[1] http://info.cancerresearchuk.org/cancerstats/types/oral/?a=5441 (accessed December 2005).
http://www.statistics.gov.uk/census 2001/pyramids(accessed March 2006)

Outcome measure (disease status)

The principal outcome measure is the incidence of periodontitis based on **person-years-at-risk** (*paragraphs 6 and 12*). Periodontitis was assessed every 2 years by the question 'Have you had professionally diagnosed periodontal disease with bone loss?'. The assessment of disease status depends on the self-report of the men and whether they have seen a dentist. To determine the accuracy of the self-reporting, the researchers took a sub-sample of individuals and compared their self-reported periodontitis status with an independent assessment made using their dental records (radiographs). There was a close correspondence between the two, indicating that in this population of health professionals, self-reporting is a valid measure of periodontitis.

Exposure measure (risk factor)

Alcohol consumption was measured in grams per day and the subjects were divided into non-drinkers and four drinking categories. This was done using a food frequency questionnaire completed by participants in 1986, 1990 and 1994, which asked about alcohol intake in the previous year (*paragraph 4*). Exposure was taken to be the average intake before the development of periodontitis, thus allowing for changes in drinking habits over time.

What are the main results?

The main results are shown in *Table 2* in the paper. There were 2125 men who developed periodontitis during the 12-year period (found by summing the second row of the table). The table shows the relative risk of developing periodontitis in each category of alcohol intake, where the comparison group is the non-drinkers.

Risk of developing periodontitis – drinkers compared with non-drinkers

There were 39 461 men in the study, and they spent a total of 406 160 person-years (found by summing the third row of *Table 2* in the paper) in the study. This means that on average each man spent just over 10 years in the study (406 160 ÷ 39 461). There were 2125 men who developed periodontitis during the 12-year period, so the incidence rate is 5.2 per 1000 person-years [(2125/406 160) × 1000]. *Table 2* in the paper gives the relative risks separately for each of the alcohol intake groups compared with no drinking. In Table 6.3 we show how to calculate the relative risk for all the alcohol drinkers combined versus the non-drinkers, that is the risk of drinking some alcohol versus the risk of drinking none at all. The relative risk of 1.28 is called the **crude** or **unadjusted** estimate because it ignores any effect of possible confounding factors. It tells us that drinkers are 1.28 times more likely to develop periodontitis than non-drinkers (or the risk is increased by 28%).

Interpreting Table 2 in the paper

Although crude estimates give an overall idea of the effect of an exposure on the risk of a disease, we need to see if an excess risk persists after allowing for confounding

Table 6.3 Calculation of relative risk of periodontitis in all drinkers versus non-drinkers. Pitiphat *et al.* (2003).

| | | Drinker | | |
		No	Yes[*]	Relative risk
No. of men in study		9442	29 990	
No. of person-years (Y)	Y	85 814	320 346	
No. of new cases of periodontitis	P	373	1752	
Proportion of new cases of periodontitis per person-year	P/Y	0.0043	0.0055	
Incidence rate of periodontitis per 1000 person-years	(P/Y) × 1000	4.3	5.5	**5.5/4.3 = 1.28**

[*] Found by summing the number of men, cases and person-years in the four alcohol consumption categories in *Tables 1 and 2* in the paper.

factors. This is addressed in *Table 2* of the paper. Many papers include a similar presentation of results, so it is worth looking carefully at the elements in the table, and being clear about what they mean. Each row of relative risks gives us information about the relationship between drinking and periodontitis after adjusting for various confounders. The table shows the relative risks for each different category of alcohol intake. The relative risk for no alcohol intake (the column labelled '0' in *Table 2*) is taken as 1. Relative risks involve comparing the risk at one level of exposure with the risk at another level of exposure. Here we are comparing the risks at the various levels of alcohol intake with the no intake category; it is called the **reference group.**

Figure 6.3 shows the elements in *Table 2* of the paper and what they mean. The row titled 'Age-adjusted RR' tells us that people who drank 0.1–4.9 g/day are 1.21 times as likely as non-drinkers to get periodontitis; those who drank 5–14.9 g/day are 1.20 times as likely as non-drinkers to get periodontitis, and so on up to 1.57 times as much risk for those who drank ≥30 g/day. The confidence interval below each relative risk can be used to see if the relative risk is statistically significant. If the confidence interval does not contain 1 (the no effect value) then the increase in risk is statistically significant. Looking at each of the confidence intervals in the row, none of them contain 1, so in each of the drinking categories the increase in risk compared to not drinking alcohol is statistically significant.

Adjusting for confounders

The results presented so far suggest that drinking alcohol is associated with an increased risk of periodontitis. However, we need to consider if this link has arisen because drinkers differ from non-drinkers in other respects which affect the comparison. For example, could the increased risk really be due to smoking, because drinkers are more likely to smoke? Or could other factors be influencing the association, such

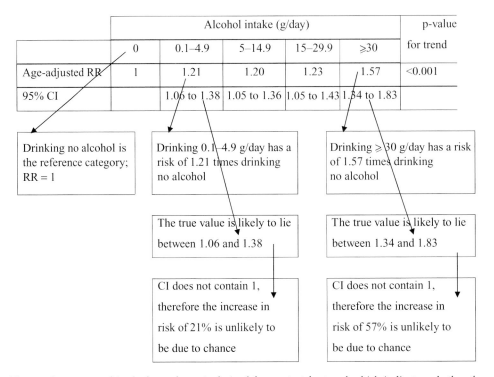

The p-value presented in the last column is derived from a test for trend which indicates whether the relative risks increase with increasing alcohol intake. It is not related to the statistical significance of the individual relative risks.

Figure 6.3 Description of the main results in *Table 2* of the paper by Pitiphat *et al.* (2003).

as drinkers being older or poorer or less physically active than non-drinkers? To illustrate how to approach this question, we focus on the result in the highest category of consumption ($\geq$30 g/day). Age is always a factor to consider in cohort studies because, for many diseases, the likelihood of having the disease increases with age. Smoking is a contributing factor in many diseases and is higher in drinkers, so it may also be a confounder here.

What is the evidence for smoking as a confounder? *Table 1* in the paper shows that, in this sample of men, smoking is associated with alcohol drinking; the proportion of current smokers clearly increases with alcohol intake. It is also well known from previous evidence that smoking is associated with periodontitis (*paragraph 23*). Therefore some or all of the risk of periodontitis that drinkers experience could actually be due to their smoking habit.

Earlier in this chapter, we showed that a confounder can be allowed for by analysing the data separately within each level of the confounder (called stratification). There are, however, more sophisticated methods of doing this; these are particularly useful when there are several factors to allow for and it becomes impractical

Table 6.4 Relative risk of periodontitis among men who drank ≥ 30 g/day compared to non-drinkers (Pitiphat *et al.*, 2003).

Risk adjusted for:	Relative risk (95% CI)
None (crude estimate)[*]	1.60 (1.37 to 1.86)
Age	1.57 (1.34 to 1.83)
Age and smoking	1.29 (1.09 to 1.53)
Age, smoking, diabetes, body mass index, physical activity, total calorie intake and calendar time	1.27 (1.08 to 1.49)

[*] Estimated using data in *Table 2*; $(282/40\,611) \div (373/85\,814) = 1.60$.

to separate and analyse the data in many small subgroups. In the current paper, the method of analysis used is **multiple logistic regression** (*paragraph 8*). This analysis provides estimates of the relative risk after it has been adjusted for particular confounders. The details of the method are not needed for the purpose of this book. What matters is that we know the relative risk has been appropriately adjusted for confounding factors which might be related to both exposure and disease.

Table 6.4 shows the relative risk of periodontitis associated with drinking ≥ 30 g/day compared with non-drinkers, after adjustment for confounders. The crude relative risk of periodontitis in heavy drinkers compared with non-drinkers is 1.60 (an excess risk of 60%). When the data are adjusted for age the relative risk result decreases only by a small amount to 1.57, indicating that the effect of age is small. When the relative risk is adjusted for both age and smoking it reduces to 1.29 (an excess risk of 29%) but most of this is due to smoking. These results show that there is some confounding effect of smoking, and perhaps half of the increased risk associated with alcohol could really be due to smoking (the crude excess risk is 60% and this reduces to 29% after allowance for age and smoking, so the difference of 31% is the excess risk that is largely due to smoking; $31/60 \approx 0.5$).

The relative risk of 1.29 has a 95% confidence interval of 1.09 to 1.53; this does not include 1 (the no effect value) so the result is statistically significant, implying that the 29% increase is unlikely to be a chance finding in this particular study. We can conclude that heavy drinking does have an effect on periodontitis even after age and smoking habits have been taken into account. Clearly, smoking is the most important confounder that has been measured here. If we look at what happens to the relative risk after it has been adjusted for a further five factors, it only decreases from 1.29 to 1.27. This final analysis shows that the association between drinking and peridontitis still holds up even when we adjust for several other potential confounders.

In summary, when investigating the effect of an exposure as a risk factor for a disease, the first step is to see if there is any association between the two (the crude relative risk). The next step is to see if the association is maintained after adjustment for other potential risk factors.

Does risk increase with increasing exposure?

If risk increases as the amount of exposure increases, this is evidence in favour of a causal link between the exposure and outcome. Does the relative risk for periodontitis increase as alcohol consumption increases? The heaviest drinking category always has the highest relative risk (*Table 2*). The researchers have performed a 'test for trend' (*paragraph 10* and *Table 2*) which is similar to a linear regression between alcohol intake and risk of periodontitis. This was done to determine whether the relative risk increased as alcohol consumption increased. The trend tests are statistically significant for the age-adjusted and age and smoking-adjusted relative risks ($p < 0.0001$ and $p = 0.02$). They indicate that even after adjustment for age and smoking the risk of periodontitis increases with increasing alcohol consumption, and this is unlikely to be due to chance.

Subgroup analysis – risk according to different types of alcohol

Analyses of risks within subsets of the data are called **subgroup analyses**. These should be interpreted with caution, partly because the number of subjects in each subgroup will be small compared to the total sample and may not be large enough to detect associations if these exist. *Table 3* in the paper shows the relative risk of developing periodontitis according to type of alcohol (beer, red wine, white wine and spirits). If we focus on the highest consumption category, all the relative risks are above 1, consistent with an increased risk. However the 95% confidence intervals include 1 suggesting the increases in risk may be chance findings. The lack of certainty in the results is shown in the wide confidence intervals. For example, the relative risk for the highest category of white wine consumption is 1.14, a 14% excess risk, and the 95% confidence interval is 0.79 to 1.66; indicating that the true change in risk could be anywhere between a 21% reduction or 66% increase in risk. Although the result is not statistically significant, we cannot conclude that white wine consumption has no effect on periodontitis. It may be that there is an effect but our sample is just too small to show it conclusively. The authors say that these subgroup analyses should be viewed with caution (*paragraph 18*), particularly because there were too few heavy drinkers in each category to give a precise estimate of the effect of consuming different types of alcohol.

How good is the evidence?

Exposure was measured before the development of disease

Men who had periodontitis at the start of the study were excluded (*paragraph 3*). This ensured that all the cases of periodontitis recorded arose during the course of the study, after alcohol intake had been measured. An exposure can only be a cause of disease if people are exposed *before* they develop the disease.

Alcohol exposure was assessed at baseline, enabling the investigators to look at consumption before the onset of disease. Possible confounders (smoking) and other characteristics (for example body mass index, physical activity) were also measured at baseline, before the development of disease (*paragraph 9*).

Frequency of measurement of disease status and exposure status

Periodontitis was assessed every 2 years (*paragraph 6*), therefore subjects were only expected to recall whether they had been diagnosed with periodontitis over the previous 2 years. If the recall period had been much longer subjects would be more likely to forget a previous diagnosis from, say, 10 years ago, and the observed incidence would be an underestimate of the true incidence.

Alcohol exposure was assessed at baseline and at three further time points (*paragraph 4*). This allowed the researchers to estimate the average alcohol intake over time. If alcohol use had only been observed once at the start of the study, the investigators would have had to assume that it remained constant during the study period.

How accurate were the measurements of disease and exposure?

All the data on exposure and the disease came from questionnaires that were completed by the subjects. It therefore relied on the accuracy with which the subjects recorded the information over the years. The possible effect of misclassification (people who do not have periodontitis but report that they do, or people who have periodontitis but report that they do not) was explored by the authors who conducted studies to validate self-reporting of periodontitis against clinical criteria (*paragraph 24*). They also state that misreporting tends to be random; this would mean that people are equally likely to over-report periodontitis as under-report it. However, misreporting is not always random because, for example, it is known that smokers and alcohol drinkers tend to under-report their consumption.

Sample size and number of cases

The study was based on a large sample of men, 39 461, and a long study period, 12 years. This provided a relatively large number of cases (people with the disease) on which to base the results and conclusions. For a cohort study to be successful, follow-up has to be long enough to allow a sufficient number of people to develop the disease.

Lost to follow-up

If a large number of subjects are lost during follow-up, this can affect the results. Bias arises if the reasons for dropping out are connected with either the outcome or the exposure. For example, in any study of alcohol consumption it is possible that the heaviest drinkers are less likely to complete the study because of alcohol-related problems. This could mean that we underestimate the effect of alcohol consumption. It is possible to check for this sort of bias by looking at whether the proportion of drop-outs is the same in the different exposure categories (for example in drinkers and non-drinkers).

One reason for basing a cohort study on health professionals is that they have to be registered with their professional body, therefore they are easier to keep in contact with than people in other occupations. Subjects in this study had to be contacted regularly during a 12-year period. The authors do not report the extent of loss to follow-up but it is likely to have been small because the subjects were easy to trace.

Confounding

Confounding can be dealt with at the design stage of a study or in the statistical analysis. Two potential confounders in this study were gender and socio-economic status and the effects of these were avoided by recruiting only one gender (men) who were all of similar socio-economic status (health professionals) (*paragraph 2*). Not every potential confounder can be allowed for in the selection of the sample, because this would make recruitment too restrictive; other confounders can be adjusted for in the statistical analysis. At the start of a cohort study, decisions about what measurements to include are based on first ensuring that known risk factors for which evidence already exists are included, and then adding other factors which might be risk factors, but for which evidence has not yet been obtained. Here, age, smoking and diabetes are known risk factors for periodontitis. Physical activity, body mass index and total calories are all related to general health and could be risk factors. Even after allowing for the confounders that have been measured, there may still be some that are as yet unknown. It is possible that part of the observed association could be due to these unknown factors.

Adjustment was made for a major confounder (smoking) and the association between drinking and periodontitis remained statistically significant and clinically important. The other potential confounders had little effect on the relative risk (*Table 2* in the paper). In the discussion the authors draw attention to one possible confounder that was not measured in the study, oral hygiene. There is evidence from other research that alcohol drinkers have poorer oral hygiene than non-drinkers (*paragraph 21*), and we know that oral hygiene is associated with periodontitis. Because oral hygiene is associated with both exposure (drinking) and outcome it might, therefore, be a confounder and account for part of the association between periodontitis and drinking. Although information on oral hygiene practice was not collected for the whole cohort, it was looked at in a subsample who were found to have good oral hygiene. This is expected given that all the subjects in the study were health professionals, of whom 58% were dentists (*paragraph 2*). The authors conclude that oral hygiene is unlikely to confound the effect of alcohol in this cohort (*paragraph 21*).

Residual confounding (*paragraph 23*) occurs when the statistical techniques used to adjust for a confounder may not completely remove its effect, so even after adjustment there is still a small influence of the confounder (hence the term residual confounding). This situation can occur when the relation between the confounder and either the disease of interest or exposure is very strong. The authors have addressed this by restricting the data to non-smokers only (in whom there can be no residual effect of smoking), and shown that the association between alcohol and periodontitis remains (*paragraphs 12 and 23*).

Confounding is common in observational studies. When we find an association and are trying to decide if it might be causal, we need first to assure ourselves that the association is maintained after adjustment for other factors that might also explain the results.

Box 6.1

Features of causality

1 The exposure must come before the onset of disease (time sequence)
2 There is an association between exposure and the disease that is unlikely to be due to chance
3 There is a dose–response relationship between exposure and risk
4 The association between the exposure and disease remains after adjustment for confounders
5 The risk of the disease reduces if the exposure is removed (reversibility)
6 The results of different studies are consistent
7 It is biologically plausible that the exposure causes the disease (evidence for this could come from human or animal studies)

Features of causality

When an association is found between an exposure and an outcome, this does not necessarily imply that the exposure causes the outcome. In the example above, alcohol is clearly associated with periodontitis, but what further evidence would support the case for alcohol being a *cause* of periodontitis? The features listed in Box 6.1 strengthen the proposition that an association is causal. How do these criteria apply to the association between alcohol consumption and periodontitis?

(1) *The exposure must come before the onset of disease (time sequence).* For a risk factor to be a cause of disease a person must be exposed to it before developing the disease. This is a cohort study that excluded people who already had periodontitis at the start and only included those who developed periodontitis during the course of the study. The incident risk of periodontitis is compared with alcohol consumption during the study prior to diagnosis, so the exposure had occurred before the development of the disease.

(2) *There is an association between exposure and the disease that is unlikely to be due to chance.* In this study there is an increased risk of periodontitis for all categories of drinking, and these increases are statistically significant.

(3) *There is a dose–response relation between exposure and risk.* As alcohol consumption increases the risk of periodontitis rises and this trend is statistically significant.

(4) *The association between the exposure and disease remains after adjustment for confounders.* After the relative risks are adjusted for age and smoking, and other potential confounders (*Table 2* in the paper) they are still greater than 1 and statistically significant.

(5) *The risk of the disease reduces if the exposure is removed (reversibility).* A well-known example of this is that lifelong smokers who give up at the age of 50 halve their chance of dying from smoking-related diseases. In the study on alcohol and periodontitis

it would be possible to look at reversibility by seeing whether people who gave up alcohol during the course of the study had a lower risk of developing periodontitis than those who continued drinking. The authors of the current study have not reported this, possibly because the number of people who gave up alcohol was too small to provide a reliable answer.

(6) *The results are consistent across different studies.* Different studies are based on different groups of people, so if the reported results on a particular association are consistent between studies this provides good evidence of an underlying effect. The current study was based on US male health professionals aged 40–75 years but several other observational studies have been done. These studies have included men and women from the general population, subjects aged below 40 years and subjects from several countries, including Japan, China, the USA and Finland. The studies all reported that alcohol users had a higher risk of periodontitis, confirming that the association between alcohol and periodontitis is consistent across different studies (*paragraphs 1, 16, 17*).

(7) *It is biologically plausible that the exposure causes the disease.* Other studies have examined possible biological mechanisms (*paragraph 20*). Alcohol impairs neutrophil function; it may stimulate bone reabsorbtion and suppress bone turnover; it may have a direct effect on the periodontium; and high alcohol consumption increases cytokine production.

Is there a causal link between alcohol and periodontitis?

The case for a causal link between alcohol and periodontitis is well supported in several ways. The association between alcohol and periodontitis is unlikely to be due to chance; it shows a dose–response relation; it remains after adjustment for confounders; the exposure comes before the onset of disease; the effect has been shown consistently in different populations; and it is biologically plausible. All these increase the likelihood that the association is causal – that alcohol consumption causes periodontitis.

Determing whether an association is causal or not is rarely based on only one study. The case for causality is strengthened when there is epidemiological evidence from several sources, the effect is found in different groups of people, and there is evidence from biological studies.

What does the study contribute to dental practice?

Who will the results apply to?

Because the subjects are all male health professionals they may not be representative of the general population because they may have different characteristics, for example, better oral hygiene. This would be important if we were trying to assess prevalence but it is less so when we are looking for risk factors.

The study took place in the USA and similar associations have been found in other countries, so the results would probably apply in the UK. The study was based on men aged 40–75 years. Would the results be applicable to women or to people aged less than 40 years? It is biologically plausible that alcohol would also have some adverse effect in women or younger people, although the size of the increase in risk in these groups may vary.

The study clearly shows that alcohol intake is **associated** with the risk of periodontitis. Consideration of the findings and other evidence strengthens the possibility that the association is casual. Patients can be advised that alcohol consumption is likely to increase their risk of periodontal disease.

CASE–CONTROL STUDIES

Case–control studies are another type of observational study which is used to examine associations between exposures and oral disease. These are sometimes referred to as **retrospective** studies. In a cohort study we start with people who are disease-free and observe new cases of the disease over a period of time. Case–control studies start with some people who have the disease of interest and some who do not and their past history of exposure is ascertained. Figure 6.4 illustrates this. There are two major issues in the design of case–control studies:

- How were the controls selected?
- What steps have been taken to reduce bias and confounding?

Selection of controls

The controls should be representative of the population at risk of the disease. Cases and controls should be as alike as possible in everything except the exposure. Some types of control that have been used are:

- Hospital controls – treated in the same hospital as cases, but for some other condition
- Family members – spouse, sibling, cousin
- Neighbours
- People registered with the same dentist

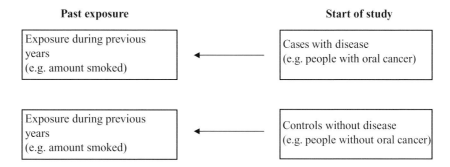

Figure 6.4 Illustration of the design of a case–control study.

Bias

Selection bias is when study subjects are chosen in such a way as to spuriously increase or decrease the magnitude of an association. This can happen if the selection criteria for controls are in some way related to exposure. In an early study undertaken by a respiratory physician to see if smoking was associated with lung cancer he compared rates of previous smoking between his lung cancer patients (cases) and patients with other respiratory illness (controls). The lung cancer patients had smoked more, but their increase in risk compared to other respiratory patients was small. This is because smoking is a cause in almost all respiratory illness, so the controls were also heavier smokers than the general population. This study therefore underestimated the effect of smoking on the risk of lung cancer.

Recall bias frequently affects the results of case–control studies, where the information on exposure comes from asking the patient to recall their past exposure and remember what they did some time ago, even several years ago. People with disease often try to find some explanation for why they contracted the disease. This can lead to a difference in recall between cases and controls, which may result in an inflated estimate of the association between the risk factor concerned and the disease.

Confounding

Known or potential confounding factors can be allowed for either at the design stage or during statistical analysis. When designing a case–control study, controls can be selected on the basis that they are similar to cases with regards to specified factors, such as age. In the statistical analysis, other confounders can be allowed for by using similar statistical techniques to those used in analysing cohort studies (for example multiple logistic regression, see section 'Adjusting for confounders' on page 123).

AN EXAMPLE OF A CASE–CONTROL STUDY

To introduce case–control studies we present an example using the following reference:

Reference: McGrother, C.W., Dugmore, C., Phillips, M.J., Raymond, N.T., Garrick, P. and Baird, W.O. Multiple sclerosis, dental caries and fillings: a case–control study. *Br Dent J* 1999; **187**:261–264.

Only the Abstract and the Methods section have been reproduced rather than the complete paper (see pp. 152–153).

What is the aim of the study?

The aim is to examine the association between multiple sclerosis, dental caries and type of fillings. The study was prompted by previous reports that people with multiple sclerosis were 'cured' when their amalgam fillings were replaced and the possibility that amalgam fillings led to raised mercury levels in the body, which could be a risk factor for multiple sclerosis.

What is the main outcome measure?

The presence or absence of multiple sclerosis. In a case–control study the outcome measure is defined by the disease of the cases.

What are the exposure measures?

The number of decayed, missing and filled teeth (DMFT) was the principal exposure measure. The number of teeth filled with amalgam and with non-amalgam were also recorded, as were blood concentrations of mercury and lead.

All cases and controls had a dental examination at home. The following measurements and information were obtained (*paragraphs 3–5*):

- DMFT index
- Number of teeth filled with amalgam or with non-amalgam
- An assessment of dental hygiene
- Demographics (for example home owner, socio-economic group)
- Urine sample for analysis of mercury levels
- Blood sample for analysis of mercury and lead levels

How was the study conducted?

Selection of cases

The cases, people with multiple sclerosis, were identified from a regional hospital discharge database in Leicestershire UK, (*paragraph 1*). It is essential to have standard and accepted criteria for diagnosing the disease and identifying cases, particularly for diseases where a range of diagnostic methods may be used. In this study four of the selection criteria related to diagnosis were:

- International Classification of Diseases (ICD) code 340 on the hospital register
- Neurological abnormalities on examination
- Thought by a neurologist to have probable or definite multiple sclerosis
- Two further diagnostic criteria recommended by Shumacher

Selection of controls

The controls, people without multiple sclerosis, were **matched** with the cases (*paragraph 2*). Matching is a way of reducing the effect of known confounders and involves selecting controls who are similar to cases with regard to specific characteristics. To do this, a control (or several controls) is identified who has characteristics that match those of a case as closely as possible. In the current study, the researchers aimed to identify four controls for each case, and they had to have the following characteristics:

- Female
- White
- Were within 2.5 years of the age of the case
- Were with the same general practitioner
- Did not have any known neurological disorders

Having several controls for each case increases the power of the study to detect an association.

There were 329 women with multiple sclerosis aged 25–65 years who were identified from the computerised admissions system. After applying the criteria for selection (see above), 49 cases remained of whom 39 agreed to take part in the study, a response rate of 81%. Of the 105 controls approached, 62 agreed to participate: a response rate of 59%.

What are the main results?

In case–control studies, the measure of the association between exposure and the risk of disease is called the **odds ratio** (analogous to relative risk in cohort studies). Odds are commonly used in gambling. For example a bookmaker may offer odds of 20 to 1 (sometimes written 20:1 or 20/1) that England will win the World Cup. This means that the bookmaker thinks the probability that England will lose the cup is 20 times the probability that England will win. In dentistry, it is usually the odds of having a disease that is of interest, and the number of people with disease is compared with the number of people without disease. For example, if the chance of having a disease is 2 in 7 then there will be two people with the disease for every five without; the odds are therefore 2:5. In the same way that a relative risk is defined as the ratio of two proportions, an odds ratio is the ratio of the odds of having the disease in one exposure group to the odds in another group (see appendix II). This calculation is illustrated using hypothetical data based on the association between multiple sclerosis and social class (Table 6.5).

An **odds ratio** can usually be interpreted in a similar way to a relative risk. Although the odds ratio and relative risk are calculated differently, if the disease is not common, the odds ratio is close to the relative risk.

Table 6.6 summarises the main results from the paper. The odds ratios were based on the increase in risk associated with one decayed, missing or filled tooth (DMFT); they were obtained from a logistic regression (*paragraph 6*). In the current study, the odds ratio associated with DMFT is 1.09. This means that for an *increase of one tooth with caries*, there is an increase of 9% in the risk of having multiple sclerosis. This result is just statistically significant (p-value = 0.049). We can use the result to estimate the increase in risk for any increase in DMFT*. For example, for an increase of 5 DMFT, the odds ratio is 1.54 (i.e. a 54% increase in risk). In the paper, the authors noted that the

---

* The odds ratio associated with an increase of n teeth is $(1.09)^n$.

Table 6.5 Hypothetical data to illustrate how to calculate an odds ratio. The data are based on the association between multiple sclerosis and social class.

	Cases with disease	Controls without disease	Odds of being a case in social class III and IV compared with social class I and II
Social class III and IV	$a = 10$	$b = 25$	$10/25 = 0.4$
Social class I and II	$c = 30$	$d = 35$	$30/35 = 0.86$
Total	40	60	

Odds ratio is

$$\frac{10/25}{30/35} = \frac{10 \times 35}{25 \times 30} = 0.47$$

$$\frac{a/b}{c/d} = \frac{a \times d}{c \times b}$$

difference in DMFT between cases and controls was 2.24, i.e. subjects with multiple sclerosis had, on average, 2.24 extra decayed, missing or filled teeth compared with unaffected controls. Such a difference would be associated with an odds ratio of 1.21 ($1.09^{2.24}$ or a 21% increase in risk). There was no association between the risk of having multiple sclerosis and amalgam fillings (odds ratio 0.96; close to the no effect value of 1). Although there seemed to be evidence of an association with non-amalgam fillings (odds ratio 1.27), the authors said this result was due to four cases only, whose fillings had been completely replaced. This is a problem with small studies – unusual characteristics of a few subjects can have a marked effect on the results.

Table 6.6 Main results on the association between caries and amalgam fillings and the risk of having multiple sclerosis from the paper by McGrother et al. (1999).

	Difference between the mean number of affected teeth (cases − controls)	Odds ratio for having multiple sclerosis associated with one extra affected tooth (95% CI)	p-value for the odds ratio
Number of DMFT*	2.24	1.09 (1.00 to 1.18)	0.049
Number of teeth filled with amalgam	−0.82	0.96 (0.87 to 1.06)	0.40
Number of teeth filled with non-amalgam	1.53	1.27 (1.04 to 1.54)	0.017

* Called DMFT index in the *Table 2* in the paper. DMFT, decayed, missing or filled teeth.

Table 6.7   Mercury and lead levels in cases and controls in the study by McGrother *et al.* (1999).

Measurement	Mean levels			
	Cases	**Controls**	**Difference**	**p-value**
Urinary mercury (creatinine ratio)				
All subjects	1.90	2.74	−0.84	0.20
Excluding outliers	1.65	1.83	−0.18	0.51
Blood mercury (nmol/l)	8.91	8.58	0.33	0.81
Blood lead (nmol/l)	0.33	0.36	−0.03	0.42

The authors also reported results on the mercury and lead levels of cases and controls, because a difference in mercury levels would lend support to the hypothesis that amalgam fillings increase the risk of developing multiple sclerosis. Table 6.7 shows that there was no evidence that either mercury or lead levels differed between cases and controls.

How good is the evidence?

The authors conclude that there is evidence for an association between caries and multiple sclerosis, but it is not strong; the effect size was small and the p-value was just under 0.05. There are other aspects of how the study was conducted and analysed that we need to take into account when considering the strength of the evidence from this study.

Selection bias

The percentage of cases who agreed to participate was higher than that for controls (81% versus 59%). The results could, therefore, be affected by selection bias. Indeed the authors state that 'The difference in dental caries rates found could be explained if a bias had operated to select a control group with artificially low levels of dental caries.'

Size of study

The study was relatively small, only 39 cases, and it was not possible to obtain four controls for each case as intended. This makes it difficult to detect a small association if one really exists.

Confounders

The researchers adjusted for a possible confounder, social class, and found that the results did not change the odds ratio. There could also be unknown confounders. An odds ratio of 1.09, if adjusted for an important confounder, could easily reduce to 1.0 (no effect).

Did exposure come before onset of disease?

It is not possible to infer from this study whether the exposure (dental caries) came before or after the onset of the disease (multiple sclerosis). It could be, for example, that people with multiple sclerosis have more caries simply because they have difficulty cleaning their teeth. Determining that exposure came before the disease is frequently a problem with case–control studies. This is because they are designed on the basis of current disease status, then their exposure is measured over some period in the past.

The study provided some evidence that caries may be a risk factor for multiple sclerosis, but no evidence of an association with having amalgam fillings. We can also consider the evidence for dental caries as a **cause** of multiple sclerosis. A summary of each of the features of causality in this particular situation is provided in Box 6.2.

Box 6.2

Feature of causality		Comment
There is an association between exposure and the disease that is unlikely to be due to chance	Yes	A small increased risk associated with dental caries was reported that was just statistically significant
There is a dose–response relation between exposure and risk	Not known	No results on dose–response were reported
The association between the exposure and disease remains after adjustment for confounders	Yes	However, only one confounder was adjusted for, there could be others
The exposure must come before the onset of disease (time sequence)	Not known	It is not possible to tell whether dental caries came before the onset of multiple sclerosis
The results are consistent between different studies	No	Some studies have reported an association but others have not
The risk of the disease should reduce if the exposure is removed (reversibility)	Not known	Cannot determine this from the study
There is biological plausibility (this could come from human or animal studies)	Weak	There is some evidence that periodontal disease is associated with certain diseases (such as heart disease), so it may be associated with multiple sclerosis

What does the study contribute to dental practice?

Because the study found no evidence of an association between amalgam fillings and the risk of developing multiple sclerosis, there is no reason to change practice.

Key points

- The rate of occurrence is a measure of how many new events occur during a specified period of time.
- Cohort and case–control studies are used to investigate the association between a risk factor (exposure) and a disease (outcome).
- A confounding factor distorts the relationship between the exposure and the outcome. It can either obscure the relationship of interest or spuriously create one.
- A factor can only be a confounder if it is associated with both the exposure of interest and the disease.
- Analysis of observational studies should allow for confounding factors to see if the association is maintained; does the relative risk (or other comparison) change materially after adjustment for confounders?
- Association does not mean that an exposure and outcome are causally related.
- There are several accepted features that strengthen the proposition that an association is causal.

Appendix I is a table that could be completed when reading an observational study (e.g. using the cohort study by Pitiphat *et al.*). The table provides some guidelines for assessing such studies. If all the points cannot be completely addressed it does not necessarily mean that the conclusions are not valid or useful.

Acknowledgements

We are grateful to the *Journal of Dental Research* (published by the International and American Associations of Dental Research) and the *British Dental Journal* (published by Macmillan) for kindly giving permission to reproduce the articles on a cohort and case–control study in chapter.

Exercise

The following is a summary of a published cohort study.

Reference: Bruno-Ambrosius, K., Swanholm, G. and Twetman, S. Eating habits, smoking and toothbrushing in relation to dental caries: a 3-year study in Swedish female teenagers. *Int J Paediatr Dent* 2005;**15**:190–196.

What is the aim of the study? To examine the effect of eating habits, smoking and toothbrushing on caries development.

Table 6.8 Odds ratios for developing caries (an increase of ≥1 DMFS during the 3-year study period) associated with several risk factors in the study by Bruno-Ambrosius *et al.*

Risk factor	Exposure group (N = number of subjects)	Reference group (N = number of subjects)	Odds ratio for having an increase of ≥1 DMFS (95% CI)
Breakfast before school	Does not have breakfast every day N = 23	Has breakfast every day N = 139	4.9 (1.4 to 17.3)
School lunch	Does not have lunch every day N = 14	Has lunch every day N = 148	1.6 (0.5 to 5.4)
Evening meal at home	Does not have dinner every day N = 41	Has dinner every day for 6 or 7 days per week N = 121	2.8 (1.3 to 6.4)
Snacks and sweets	Eats snacks and sweets several times a day N = 8	Never or seldom eats snacks and sweets, or if so it is daily or several times per week N = 154	5.5 (0.7 to 46.1)
Soft drinks or juice	Drinks soft drinks/juice several times a day N = 26	Never or seldom drinks soft drinks/juice, or if so it is daily or several times per week N = 136	1.2 (0.5 to 2.9)
Smoking	Smokes cigarettes for ≥3 days per week N = 14	Non-smoker or smokes cigarettes ≤2 days per week N = 148	4.1 (1.0 to 8.9)

How was the study conducted? The cohort included all girls aged 12 years who were listed as recall patients in the two public health dental clinics in Falkenberg (a small town on the west coast of Sweden). A questionnaire that recorded details of eating, smoking and toothbrushing was given at the start of the study and repeated every four months for three years. Subjects had a thorough dental examination at the start of the study and three years later. A total of 185 girls agreed to take part in the study and had a baseline dental examination, and 162 attended the three-year dental examination.

What was the outcome measure? Caries was measured by the number of decayed, missing or filled surfaces (DMFS) during a detailed dental examination. The increase in DMFS (DMFS at three years minus DMFS at baseline) was used as the outcome measure in the statistical analysis. Subjects were divided into two groups: those who had no increase in DMFS during the three-year study period and those who had at least one DMFS during the three years.

What was the exposure? Several risk factors were examined:
- Having breakfast at home before going to school
- Having school lunch
- Having dinner or an evening meal at home
- Frequency of consumption of snacks and sweets (divided into four categories: never or very seldom; several times a week; daily; several times a day)
- Frequency of consumption of soft drinks or juice (divided into four categories: never or very seldom; several times a week; daily; several times a day)
- Cigarette smoking

What are the main results? Table 6.8 summarises the main results.

Questions

(1) What is an advantage of only including girls aged 12 years old in the study? What are an advantage and disadvantage of only including subjects from this one small town?

(2) What is the proportion who were lost to follow-up?

(3) The measure of disease status is the increase in DMFS observed between baseline and the 3-year dental examination. Is this an acceptable measure?

(4) In Table 6.8, which associations are statistically significant and which are not?

(5) Interpret the results associated with having breakfast.

(6) The reference group for 'breakfast before school' was those children who had breakfast every day. What would the odds ratio and 95% confidence interval be if the reference group had been taken as those children who did not have breakfast every day?

(7) Explain how eating snacks and sweets could be a confounding factor when looking at the association between having breakfast and developing caries.

(8) Interpret the result associated with eating snacks and sweets. If you think the result is not statistically significant explain why.

(9) Comment on the choice of reference group and exposure group for consumption of soft drinks/juice. How might these choices affect the observed odds ratios?

(10) From this study, can you infer that missing meals (breakfast and dinner) is a cause of caries? What other evidence would help decide this?

Answers on pp. 215–217

APPENDIX I. GUIDELINES FOR THE APPRAISAL OF AN OBSERVATIONAL STUDY USING THE COHORT STUDY BY PITIPHAT *ET AL.* (2003)

Question	Comments
1. What type of study was this?	Cohort
2. Selection of subjects	

(a) Cohort: how were subjects selected?
    Case-control: how were the cases selected?
            how were the controls selected?
	Male health professionals aged 40–75

(b) Is there a sufficient number of subjects to answer the main question?	Yes; 2125 cases of periodontitis among 51 529 men
3. Bias Were there any biases that could arise from the way the study was conducted?	
(a) Selection bias	Probably not
(b) Recall bias	No
(c) Respondent bias	No
(d) Others	
4. Assessment of disease and exposure	
(a) What exactly is the disease of interest?	Periodontitis
(b) Were diagnoses made or confirmed using standard criteria?	Yes
(c) What are the main exposure(s) of interest?	Alcohol
(d) How were the exposures measured?	Average daily intake of alcohol by questionnaire every 2 years
(e) What are the important confounders?	Smoking
(f) Are there any confounders that the researchers have not included?	Oral hygiene
(g) Is there anything about the way the disease or exposure(s) were measured that could adversely affect the results?	Probably not
(h) (Cohort studies only) Were many subjects lost to follow-up? If so, did this differ between subjects who were exposed and unexposed to the factor of interest?	Probably not

(*continued*)

Question	Comments
5. Results	
(a) What is the size of the association between the disease and exposure(s)?	Relative risk in highest alcohol intake group was 1.29
(b) Is it clinically important?	Yes
(c) What is the 95% CI (the range of estimate of the true effect)?	1.09 to 1.53
(d) Are the results likely to be due to chance?	No
(e) Have the results been adjusted for confounding?	Yes
(f) Do the associations remain after confounding (effect size, 95% CI and p-value)?	Yes
6. Is there other evidence for causality?	
(a) Exposure came before the onset of disease	Yes
(b) Risk increases with increasing (or decreasing) exposure	Yes
(c) Results are consistent with other studies	Yes
(d) If the exposure is removed the risk reduces	Cannot tell from this study
(e) The association is biologically plausible	Yes
7. The effect on dental practice	
(a) Are the study subjects similar to your population?	Results likely to apply to both adult males and females
(b) If not, is there any reason why the results of the study would not be applicable to your population?	
(c) What are the implications of this and other studies on the management of your patients, with regard to:	
Prevention?	Heavy drinkers advised to reduce intake
Diagnosis?	Take care to investigate periodontitis in patients known to have high alcohol intake
Treatment?	Patients diagnosed with periodontitis who drink heavily advised to reduce intake/stop

APPENDIX II. CALCULATION OF ODDS, RISK, ODDS RATIO AND RELATIVE RISK

	With disease	Without disease	Odds	Risk
Exposed	a	b	a/d	a/a+b
Unexposed	c	d	c/d	c/c+d
Summary measure			Odds ratio is a/b ÷ c/d	Relative risk is a/a+b ÷ c/c+d

The odds of having disease if subject is exposed is a/b
The odds of having disease if the subject is unexposed is c/d
The **odds ratio** is then found by taking the ratio of the two odds.

The risk of having disease if the subject is exposed is a/a+b
The risk of having disease if the subject is unexposed is c/c+d
The **relative risk (or risk ratio)** is then found by taking the ratio of the two risks.

The relative risk is used to describe the association between an exposure and an outcome in cohort studies. In case–control studies the odds ratio is used rather than the relative risk. The odds ratio is a measure that has a similar interpretation to a relative risk, but is calculated slightly differently. The Table shows how the two are estimated. The relative risk and odds ratio are not necessarily the same numerically. However, if the disease is rare then the odds ratio is close to the relative risk.

RESEARCH REPORTS
Clinical

Alcohol Consumption Increases Periodontitis Risk

W. Pitiphat[1*,2,3,] **A.T. Merchant**[1,2,4,] **E.B. Rimm**[2,4,5,] **and K.J. Joshipura**[1,2]

[1]Department of Oral Health Policy & Epidemiology, Harvard School of Dental Medicine, 188 Longwood Avenue, Boston, MA 02115, USA; [2]Department of Epidemiology, Harvard School of Public Health, Boston, MA, USA; [3]Department of Community Dentistry, Faculty of Dentistry, Khon Kaen University, Khon Kaen, Thailand; [4]Department of Nutrition, Harvard School of Public Health, Boston, MA, USA; and [5]The Channing Laboratory, Department of Medicine, Harvard Medical School and Brigham and Women's Hospital, Boston, MA, USA; *corresponding author, waranuch@post.harvard.edu

J Dent Res 82(7):509–513, 2003

ABSTRACT

Alcohol consumption impairs neutrophil, macrophage, and T-cell functions, increasing the likelihood of infections. We examined the association between alcohol consumption and periodontitis, prospectively, among 39,461 male health professionals aged 40 to 75 years and free of periodontitis at the start of follow-up. Alcohol intake was assessed at baseline and updated every 4 years by a food-frequency questionnaire. Periodontal disease status was self-reported and validated against radiographs. Multivariate analysis was adjusted for age, smoking, diabetes, body-mass index, physical activity, time period, and caloric intake. During 406,160 person-years of follow-up, there were 2125 cases of periodontitis. Compared with non-drinkers, the relative risk (95% confidence interval) among men reporting usual alcohol intake of 0.1–4.9 g/day was 1.24 (1.09, 1.42); 5.0 to 14.9 g/day, 1.18 (1.04, 1.35); 15 to 29.9 g/day, 1.18 (1.01, 1.38); and ≥30 g/day, 1.27 (1.08, 1.49). The results suggest that alcohol consumption is an independent modifiable risk factor for periodontitis.

KEY WORDS: alcohol drinking, epidemiology, periodontal diseases, periodontitis.

Received August 15, 2002; Last revision February 20, 2003; Accepted April 2, 2003

INTRODUCTION

Alcohol impairs neutrophil, macrophage, and T-cell functions, increasing the likelihood of infections (Szabo, 1999), possibly raising the risk of periodontitis. Despite the plausible mechanisms, information relating alcohol consumption to periodontitis risk is sparse. Previous cross-sectional (Sakki *et al.*, 1995; Shizukuishi *et al.*, 1998; Tezal *et al.*, 2001) and case-control (Pan *et al.*, 1998) studies have shown positive associations between alcohol use and periodontal disease; however, prospective data are not yet available. Furthermore, only one study has assessed the effects of different types of alcohol on the risk of periodontal disease (Tezal *et al.*, 2001). We therefore examined prospectively the association between alcohol consumption and periodontitis among men who participated in the Health Professionals Follow-up Study (HPFS).

MATERIALS & METHODS

Study Population

The HPFS is a prospective study of 51,529 male health professionals aged 40–75 years in 1986. The cohort included dentists (58%), veterinarians (20%), pharmacists (8%), optometrists (7%), osteopathic physicians (4%), and podiatrists (3%). Incident diseases and updated exposures were ascertained with biennial questionnaires. Responses to the questionnaires constituted informed consent to a protocol that was approved by the Institutional Review Board at Harvard School of Public Health.

We excluded men who were deceased (n = 4), reported periodontitis (n = 8955), reported myocardial infarction or stroke (n = 1884), or provided inadequate dietary information (n = 1225) in 1986, leaving 39,461 men eligible for follow-up.

Journal paper

Assessment of Alcohol Consumption

4 We estimated alcohol intake during the previous year from a semi-quantitative food-frequency questionnaire (FFQ), sent to the participants in 1986, 1990, and 1994. The FFQ included questions about how often, on average, the men consumed beer (1 bottle or can), wine (4-oz glass), and liquor (1 drink or shot) in the past year. For each of these items, the participants could select 1 of 9 responses, ranging from never or less than once/month to ≥6 times/day. The alcohol content is estimated to be 12.8 g for a bottle of beer, 11.0 g for a glass of wine, and 14.0 g for a drink of liquor. We calculated total alcohol consumption in grams by summing the beverage-specific product of the average daily consumption of beer, wine, and liquor and the alcohol content of that beverage.

5 We evaluated the validity of the FFQ in a random sample of 136 men living in the Boston area (Giovannucci *et al.*, 1991). Intake of alcohol reported over the previous year by the FFQ correlated highly with intake assessed by diet records completed over this period (Spearman r = 0.86, p < 0.001).

Assessment of Periodontitis

6 We assessed periodontitis every 2 yrs from 1986 to 1998 by a question, "Have you had professionally diagnosed periodontal disease with bone loss?" The positive and negative predictive values of self-report compared with radiographs (assessed in a subsample) were 76% and 74% among dentists (Joshipura *et al.*, 1996) and 83% and 69% for other health professionals (Joshipura *et al.*, 2002).

Statistical Analysis

7 Participants contributed person-time from the date of return of the baseline questionnaire to the occurrence of periodontitis, death from any cause, or December 31, 1998, whichever came first. Men who reported periodontitis on previous questionnaires were excluded from subsequent follow-up; thus, each participant could contribute only one end point.

8 We used multivariate pooled logistic regression (D'Agostino *et al.*, 1990) with two-year time intervals to approximate the Cox proportional hazards model. For the primary analyses, we modeled periodontitis risk and cumulatively averaged (Hu *et al.*, 1999) alcohol consumption. In this analysis, if a person had angina, coronary artery bypass graft surgery, myocardial infarction, stroke, cancer, or asthma, we stopped updating his alcohol intake, because he might have changed consumption as a result of the event, and it may not reflect long-term intake. In additional analyses, we related incidence of periodontitis to intake of alcohol at baseline and to the most recent intake.

9 The multivariate models adjusted for age, time period, smoking, diabetes, body mass index (BMI), physical activity (metabolic equivalents/wk), and total calories. Time-varying covariates including age, smoking, diabetes, physical activity, BMI, and total calories were updated every 2 yrs, because most recent status may be more relevant to the disease. We updated physical activity by using the cumulative average of activities during the period of follow-up to best represent long-term physical activity levels of individuals, and it reduced measurement error (Hu *et al.*, 1999). We adjusted for energy as a surrogate measure of metabolic efficiency and the thermogenic effects of foods, which may be a potential source of residual confounding.

10 The presence of a linear trend in relative risk (RR) across alcohol categories was tested with the medians within each category as an ordinal variable. We also conducted analyses separately among non-smokers and among participants who reported unchanged drinking habits during follow-up. To examine the presence of interactions, we performed the analyses stratified by age, smoking, and BMI. We used likelihood ratio tests to compare models with and without the interaction terms. All reported *p*-values are two-sided.

RESULTS

11 In this cohort, most participants (52%) had low-to-moderate alcohol consumption (0.1–14.9 g/day). Compared with men who reported drinking no alcohol, men who reported any regular alcohol intake were more likely to be smokers, were more

Table 1 Baseline Characteristics, According to Level of Alcohol Intake, among Men Free of Periodontitis in 1986[a], The Health Professionals Follow-up Study

Characteristics	Alcohol Intake (g/day)				
	0	0.1–4.9	5–14.9	15–29.9	≥30
Number (%)	9442 (24.0)	9592 (24.3)	10786 (27.4)	5174(13.1)	4438(11.3)
Mean age (yrs)	53.9	52.8	53.3	53.4	54.9
Currently smoking (%)	9.8	11.0	11.8	12.0	22.4
Mean body mass index (kg/m^2)	25.6	25.5	25.4	25.3	25.6
Physical activity (MET/week)	18.7	20.5	23.1	24.1	21.3
Diabetes (%)	4.2	2.3	1.5	1.3	2.1
Average caloric intake/day (kcal)	1930	1934	1967	2083	2223

[a] Excluding 29 men who did not give information on alcohol intake in 1986.
[b] MET, metabolic equivalent.

physically active, consumed more calories, and were less likely to be diabetic (Table 1).

During 406,160 person-years of follow-up, 2125 participants reported periodontitis for the first time. Crude incidence of periodontitis was 4.3 *per* 1000 person-years among non-drinkers and varied from 5.2 to 6.9 *per* 1000 person-years among drinkers (Table 2). After adjustment for age, men who drank alcohol were at higher risk of periodontal disease compared with non-drinkers. Further adjustment for smoking slightly attenuated

this association. There was a positive association between alcohol intake and periodontitis across all categories of intake after simultaneous adjustment for age, smoking, diabetes, BMI, physical activity, and total calories. Compared with non-drinkers, the multivariate RR among men reporting usual alcohol intake of 0.1-4.9 g/day was 1.24 (95% confidence interval [CI], 1.09, 1.42); and for ≥30 g/day, 1.27 (95% CI, 1.08, 1.49). Further analyses restricted to never-smokers (800 cases) and to participants who reported unchanged drinking habits (1823

Table 2 Relative Risk of Periodontitis According to Level of Alcohol Intake, Health Professionals Follow-up Study, 1986–1998

	Alcohol Intake (g/day)[a]					p for Trend[b]
	0	0.1–4.9	5–14.9	15–29.9	>30	
Median intake, g/day	0.0	2.1	9.3	19.6	39.7	
Number of cases	373	573	591	306	282	
Person-yrs	85,814	109,368	113,361	57,006	40,611	
Age-adjusted RR[c]	1.0	1.21	1.20	1.23	1.57	<0.001
95% CI[c]		1.06, 1.38	1.05,1.36	1.05, 1.43	1.34, 1.83	
Age- and smoking-adjusted RR	1.0	1.18	1.14	1.14	1.29	0.02
95% CI		1.03, 1.34	1.00, 1.30	0.97,1.33	1.09, 1.53	
Multivariate RR[d]	1.0	1.24	1.18	1.18	1.27	0.09
95% CI		1.09, 1.42	1.04, 1.35	1.01, 1.38	1.08, 1.49	

[a] For average intake during follow-up. A two-year period is adjusted in every analysis.
[b] The test for trend was calculated with median intake of alcohol in each category as a continuous variable.
[c] RR, relative risk; CI, confidence interval.
[d] The multivariate model adjusted for age (in five-year categories), smoking (never smoked, formerly smoked, or currently smoked fewer than 15, 15–24, or ≥25 cigarettes/day), diabetes mellitus (yes, no), body mass index (<21.0, 21.0–22.9, 23.0- < 24.9, 25.0–29.9, and 30.0 kg/m^2), physical activity (metabolic equivalent quintiles), total calories, and calendar time (two-year intervals).

Table 3 Relative Risk of Periodontitis by Baseline Consumption of Each Alcoholic Beverage, Health Professionals Follow-up Study, 1986–1998

	Alcohol Intake, Number of Drinks					
	Never or <1/mo	1–3/mo	1–4/wk	5/wk to 1/day	≥2/day	p for trend[a]
Beer						
Number of cases	875	413	538	161	103	
Multivariate RR[b]		1.04	0.93	0.84	1.06	0.63
95% CI[b]	1.0	0.91, 1.18	0.82, 1.06	0.70, 1.00	0.86, 1.31	
White Wine						
Number of cases	872	536	542	100	31	
Multivariate RR		1.05	0.11	1.06	1.14	0.21
95% CI	1.0	0.92, 1.20	0.97, 1.28	0.84, 1.32	0.79, 1.66	
Red Wine						
Number of cases	1171	461	371	61	23	
Multivariate RR	1.0	1.03	1.07	1.16	1.50	0.05
95% CI		0.90, 1.17	0.93, 1.24	0.88, 1.52	0.98, 2.30	
Liquor						
Number of cases	905	344	445	232	178	
Multivariate RR		1.08	1.01	1.07	1.15	0.13
95% CI	1.0	0.94, 1.23	0.89, 1.15	0.91, 1.25	0.97, 1.37	

[a] The test for trend was calculated with median intake of alcohol in each category as a continuous variable.
[b] The multivariate model adjusted for age (in five-year categories), smoking (never smoked, formerly smoked, or currently smoked fewer than 15, 15–24, or ≥25 cigarettes/day), diabetes mellitus (yes, no), body mass index (<21.0, 21.0–22.9, 23.0- <24.9, 25.0–29.9, and ≥30.0 kg/m^2), physical activity (metabolic equivalent quintiles), total calories, calendar time (two-year intervals), and the other alcoholic beverages in this Table simultaneously. RR denotes relative risk; CI, confidence interval.

cases) provided similar results (data not shown). We observed no evidence of effect modification by age, smoking, and BMI (data not shown).

13   Alcohol intake assessed as a cumulative average, or as a single baseline measurement, had similar associations with periodontitis risk (Fig.). The association between the most recent alcohol intake and periodontitis risk was weaker.

14   At baseline, total alcohol intake was associated with a significantly increased risk of periodontitis across all levels of intake (p for trend = 0.03) (Fig.). When we analyzed alcohol intake by the number of drinks of beer, white wine, red wine, or liquor (each adjusted for other types of alcohol), there was no clear association with periodontitis risk (Table 3). There was a modest inverse association with periodontitis risk in the third category of beer consumption, but the trend was not significant. Men who drank 2 or more glasses of red wine a day were at increased risk for periodontitis, RR =

1.50 (95% CI, 0.98, 2.30, p for trend = 0.05). White wine and liquor consumption had no appreciable effect on periodontitis. We did not find a significant difference in the test for trend between red wine and any of the other beverages.

DISCUSSION

In this large prospective study, we found a positive 15 association between alcohol intake and periodontitis. Men who drank alcohol had an 18–27% higher risk of disease than did non-drinkers. These results were similar when base-line alcohol intake was used alone, when this measure was updated every 2 yrs with most recent reported information, or when the average intake over the follow-up period was used in the analysis. Recent intake of alcohol had the weakest association, as one may expect, since it covers the shortest induction period.

Few studies have examined the possible rela- 16 tion between alcohol intake and periodontitis.

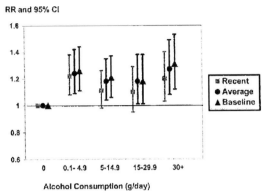

RR and 95% CI

Alcohol Consumption (g/day)

Figure. Relative risk of periodontitis according to level of alcohol intake of baseline, cumulative average intake, and recent intake, Health Professionals Follow-up Study, 1986–1998. Data are adjusted for age, smoking status, diabetes, body mass index, physical activity, total calories, and calendar time. RR denotes relative risk; 95% confidence intervals (CI) are denoted by the bars around the relative risks. The numbers of cases among those reporting baseline alcohol intake of 0.1–4.9 g/day were 528; 5.0–14.9 g/day, 589; 15–29.9 g/day, 284; for ≥30 g/day, 312; and for non-drinkers, 412. The numbers of cases among those reporting average alcohol intake of 0.1–4.9 g/day were 573; 5.0–14.9 g/day, 591; 15–29.9 g/day, 306; for ≥30 g/day, 282; and for non-drinkers, 373. The numbers of cases among those reporting recent alcohol intake of 0.1–4.9 g/day were 550; 5.0–14.9 g/day, 562; 15–29.9 g/day, 276; for ≥30 g/day, 288; and for non-drinkers, 449.

Early studies observed increased prevalence and severity of periodontal disease among patients with cirrhosis (Sandler and Stahl, 1960; Movin, 1981), and attributed this to poor oral hygiene (Movin, 1981). Other studies reported worse periodontal conditions in alcoholic patients with and without cirrhosis than in healthy subjects (Dunkley and Carson, 1968; Novacek *et al.*, 1995) and in non-alcoholic patients with cirrhosis (Novacek *et al.*, 1995). There was a significant association between alcohol consumption and periodontal disease among Japanese factory workers, but only in the bivariate analysis (Shizukuishi *et al.*, 1998). In a small study among dental patients, periodontal disease was positively associated with

indicators of alcoholism among males only, but there were only 25 female participants (Kranzler *et al.*, 1990).

A cross-sectional study of 780 Finnish men and women showed an odds ratio (OR) of 1.76 among participants who drank <7 drinks *per* 2 wks, and 2.52 among those who drank ≥7 drinks *per* 2 wks in comparison with non-drinkers, controlling for dietary habits, smoking habits, and toothbrushing frequency (Sakki *et al.*, 1995). In a case-control study in China, drinkers were 1.86 times more likely to have periodontitis than were non-drinkers (unadjusted analysis) (Pan *et al.*, 1998). Recent findings from the Erie County Study also showed a positive relationship between alcohol consumption and more severe attachment loss and gingival bleeding (Tezal *et al.*, 2001). Alcohol consumption of ≥5 drinks/wk was associated with increased attachment loss, OR of 1.36 (95% CI, 1.02,1.80), compared with consumption of <5 drinks/wk. The OR was modestly stronger (OR = 1.44; 95% CI, 1.04, 2.00) when 10 drinks/wk were used as the threshold. In the same study, wine, beer, or liquor intakes had similar associations with periodontitis risk.

We did not observe any clear pattern of association between specific beverages and periodontitis risk. High red wine intake raised the risk of periodontitis slightly more than that of the other beverages, but the result was not significant. We were somewhat limited in the beverage-specific analyses due to the limited number of cases in the heaviest drinkers; thus, the risk estimates should be interpreted with caution.

Previous studies reported a j-shaped relationship between alcohol consumption and all-cause mortality (Camargo *et al.*, 1997), driven by a reduction in risk of cardiovascular disease from moderate drinking and raised risk of cancer deaths from heavy drinking. We observed an increased risk of periodontitis with drinking any amount of alcohol. The difference in the results is due to substantially different hypothesized mechanisms to explain the association of alcohol with mortality, and with periodontitis.

Journal paper

20   Several plausible biological explanations exist for a detrimental effect of alcohol on periodontitis risk. Studies have shown that impaired neutrophil phagocytosis is associated with periodontal disease (Hart *et al.*, 1994; Van Dyke and Vaikuntam, 1994). Alcohol impairs neutrophil function, contributing to bacterial overgrowth and increased bacterial penetration (Szabo, 1999) that may lead to periodontal inflammation. Second, evidence from *in vitro* (Cheung *et al.*, 1995), animal (Farley *et al.*, 1985; Turner *et al.*, 2001), and human (Pepersack *et al.*, 1992) studies suggests that alcohol may stimulate bone resorption and suppress bone turnover. Third, alcohol may have a direct toxic effect on periodontium as with other tissues of the oropharynx (Maier *et al.*, 1994; Ogden *et al.*, 1999). Finally, moderate alcohol intake reduces monocyte production of inflammatory cytokines such as TNF-α, IL-1, and IL-6, possibly allowing for microbial proliferation (Szabo *et al.*, 1996). With higher intakes, there is more cytokine production (Szabo, 1999), and it has been shown that monocytic release of IL-1, IL-6, and TNF-α in the gingival crevice is associated with periodontitis (Offenbacher, 1996).

21   Alcohol drinking may be associated with poor oral hygiene practices (Sakki *et al.*, 1995), possibly raising periodontitis risk. Although we did not collect information on oral hygiene in the whole cohort, analysis of data from a sample of 152 men suggests that this population of health professionals had good oral hygiene. There was no significant association between oral hygiene practices and periodontal disease in this population (Merchant *et al.*, 2002), as well as in other studies (Badersten *et al.*, 1990; Machtei *et al.*, 1993; AAP, 1996). Hence, oral hygiene is unlikely to confound the effect of alcohol on periodontitis in this cohort.

22   This is the first prospective study to evaluate alcohol as a risk factor for periodontitis. The prospective design ensures temporality of the association and eliminates the possibility of recall bias. The high rate of follow-up reduced potential bias due to loss of follow-up. Men excluded due to inadequate dietary data were similar to those retained in the analysis with respect to age, smoking, physical activity, and BMI, so selection bias is unlikely. The participants are relatively homogeneous, thus minimizing confounding by race, socio-economic status, access to care, and oral hygiene practices.

23   As with any observational study, we cannot exclude the possibility of residual confounding by other habits and lifestyle factors. Since smoking is an important risk factor for periodontitis and is correlated with alcohol drinking, some degree of the observed association may be due to residual confounding by smoking. In the analysis restricted to never-smokers, the results did not change substantially, indicating that residual confounding by smoking was unlikely. In the analysis excluding participants reporting substantial change in alcohol drinking habits (possibly because of health concerns), the results were similar to the main analyses.

24   Another limitation includes the use of self-reports to assess the outcome. In such a large prospective study, it is impractical to perform clinical evaluation of periodontal disease. Our validation studies showed that self-reports of periodontitis (Joshipura *et al.*, 1996, 2002) in the HPFS population were valid. Moreover, misclassification from self-reports tends to be random, resulting in an attenuated magnitude of association; with a perfect measure of periodontitis, the association would probably be stronger.

25   In conclusion, the results support that alcohol drinking is an independent risk factor for periodontitis. Types of alcoholic beverages had no clear separate effect on periodontitis. Further research is needed to assess this association in other populations, and to determine the biological mechanisms of alcohol on periodontal disease. Health practitioners need to be aware that patients who drink may be at higher risk of periodontitis and could benefit from advice to quit smoking and maintain regular dental visits.

ACKNOWLEDGMENTS

26   This research was supported by NIH Grants CA55075, HL35464, AA11181, and DE12102.

Dr. Pitiphat is the recipient of the Royal Thai Government Scholarship. A preliminary report was presented at the 79th General Session of the International Association for Dental Research, June 27–30, 2001, Chiba, Japan.

REFERENCES

AAP (1996). Position paper: epidemiology of periodontal diseases. American Academy of Periodontology. *J Periodontol* 67:935–945.

Badersten A, Nilveus R, Egelberg J (1990). Scores of plaque, bleeding, suppuration and probing depth to predict probing attachment loss. 5 years of observation following nonsurgical periodontal therapy. *J Clin Periodontol* 17:102–107.

Camargo CA Jr, Hennekens CH, Gaziano JM, Glynn RJ, Manson JE, Stampfer MJ (1997). Prospective study of moderate alcohol consumption and mortality in US male physicians. *Arch Intern Med* 157:79–85.

Cheung RC, Gray C, Boyde A, Jones SJ (1995). Effects of ethanol on bone cells in vitro resulting in increased resorption. *Bone* 16:143–147.

D'Agostino RB, Lee ML, Belanger AJ, Cupples LA, Anderson K, Kannel WB (1990). Relation of pooled logistic regression to time dependent Cox regression analysis: the Framingham Heart Study. *Stat Med* 9:1501–1515.

Dunkley RP, Carson RM (1968). Dental requirements of the hospitalized alcoholic patient. *J Am Dent Assoc* 76:800–803.

Farley JR, Fitzsimmons R, Taylor AK, Jorch UM, Lau KH (1985). Direct effects of ethanol on bone resorption and formation in vitro. *Arch Biochem Biophys* 238:305–314.

Giovannucci E, Colditz G, Stampfer MJ, Rimm EB, Litin L, Sampson L, *et al.* (1991). The assessment of alcohol consumption by a simple self-administered questionnaire. *Am J Epidemiol* 133:810–817.

Hart TC, Shapira L, Van Dyke TE (1994), Neutrophil defects as risk factors for periodontal diseases. *J Periodontol* 65:521–529.

Hu FB, Sigal RJ, Rich-Edwards JW, Colditz GA, Solomon CG, Willett WC, *et al.* (1999). Walking compared with vigorous physical activity and risk of type 2 diabetes in women: a prospective study. *J Am Med Assoc* 282:1433–1439.

Joshipura KJ, Douglass CW, Garcia RI, Valachovic R, Willett WC (1996). Validity of a self-reported peri-odontal disease measure. *J Public Health Dent* 56: 205–212.

Joshipura KJ, Pitiphat W, Douglass CW (2002). Validation of self-reported periodontal measures among health professionals. *J Public Health Dent* 62: 115–121.

Kranzler HR, Babor TF, Goldstein L, Gold J (1990). Dental pathology and alcohol-related indicators in an outpatient clinic sample. *Community Dent Oral Epidemiol* 18:204–207.

Machtei EE, Christersson LA, Zambon JJ, Hausmann E, Grossi SG, Dunford R, *et al.* (1993). Alternative methods for screening periodontal disease in adults. *J Clin Periodontol* 20:81–87.

Maier H, Weidauer H, Zoller J, Seitz HK, Flentje M, Mall G, *et al.* (1994). Effect of chronic alcohol consumption on the morphology of the oral mucosa. *Alcohol Clin Exp Res* 18:387–391.

Merchant A, Pitiphat W, Douglass CW, Crohin C, Joshipura K (2002). Oral hygiene practices and periodontitis in health care professionals. *J Periodontol* 73:531–535.

Movin S (1981). Relationship between periodontal disease and cirrhosis of the liver in humans. *J Clin Periodontol* 8:450–458.

Novacek G, Plachetzky U, Potzi R, Lentner S, Slavicek R, Gangl A, *et al.* (1995). Dental and periodontal disease in patients with cirrhosis—role of etiology of liver disease. *J Hepatol* 22:576–582.

Offenbacher S (1996). Periodontal diseases: pathogenesis. *Ann Periodontol* 1:821–878.

Ogden GR, Wight AJ, Rice P (1999). Effect of alcohol on the oral mucosa assessed by quantitative cytomorphometry. *J Oral Pathol Med* 28:216–220.

Pan W, Zheng W, Chen S (1998). [A case-control study on risk factors of periodontitis]. *Zhonghua Liu Xing Bing Xue Za Zhi* 19:149–151.

Pepersack T, Fuss M, Otero J, Bergmann P, Valsamis J, Corvilain J (1992). Longitudinal study of bone metabolism after ethanol withdrawal in alcoholic patients. *J Bone Miner Res* 7:383–387.

Sakki TK, Knuuttila ML, Vimpari SS, Hartikainen MS (1995). Association of lifestyle with periodontal health. *Community Dent Oral Epidemiol* 23:155–158.

Sandier HC, Stahl SS (1960). Prevalence of periodontal disease in a hospitalized population. *J Dent Res* 39:439–449.

Shizukuishi S, Hayashi N, Tamagawa H, Hanioka T, Maruyama S, Takeshita T, *et al.* (1998). Lifestyle and periodontal health status of Japanese factory workers. *Ann Periodontol* 3:303–311.

Szabo G (1999). Consequences of alcohol consumption on host defence. *Alcohol Alcohol* 34:830–841.

Szabo G, Mandrekar P, Girouard L, Catalano D (1996). Regulation of human monocyte functions by acute ethanol treatment: decreased tumor necrosis factor-alpha, interleukin-1 beta and elevated interleukin-10, and transforming growth factor-beta production. *Alcohol Clin Exp Res* 20:900–907.

Tezal M, Grossi SG, Ho AW, Genco RJ (2001). The effect of alcohol consumption on periodontal disease. *J Periodontol* 72:183–189.

Turner RT, Kidder LS, Kennedy A, Evans GL, Sibonga JD (2001). Moderate alcohol consumption suppresses bone turnover in adult female rats. *J Bone Miner Res* 16:589–594.

Van Dyke TE, Vaikuntam J (1994). Neutrophil function and dysfunction in periodontal disease. *Curr Opin Periodontol* :19–27.

Journal paper

RESEARCH
epidemiology

Multiple sclerosis, dental caries and fillings: a case-control study

C. W. McGrother,[1] **C. Dugmore,**[2] **M. J. Phillips,**[3] **N. T. Raymond,**[4] **P. Garrick,**[5] **and W. O. Baird,**[6]

Objectives To investigate the association between multiple sclerosis, dental caries, amalgam fillings, body mercury and lead.

Design Matched case-control study.

Setting Leicestershire in the years 1989-1990.

Subjects Thirty-nine females with multiple sclerosis (of recent onset) were matched with 62 controls for age, sex and general practitioner.

Methods Home interview of cases and controls within which there was an assessment of the DMFT index and blood and urine mercury and lead levels.

Results The odds of being a MS case increased multiplicatively by 1.09 (95% CI 1.00,1.18) for every additional unit of DMFT index of dental caries. This represents an odds ratio of 1.213 or a 21% increase in risk of MS in relation to dental caries in this population. There was no difference between cases and controls in the number of amalgam fillings or in body mercury or lead levels. There was a significant correlation between body mercury levels and the number of teeth filled with amalgam (controls: r = +0.430, P = 0.006, cases: r = +0.596, P = 0.001).

Conclusion There was evidence of excess dental caries among MS cases compared with the controls. This finding supports the strong geographical correlation between the two diseases. A further study of this association is recommended.

Methods

Cases were identified from computerised routine hospital discharge information (Hospital Activity Analysis) for the years 1976-85, for Leicestershire, which has a population approaching one million, having established that admission of all new cases for investigation was the standard practice of local neurologists. All female admissions with the diagnosis of MS (ICD code 340) were selected because of an interest in reproductive outcomes in relation to MS and dental factors. Following the elimination of duplicate admissions and those aged less than 25 years or more than 65 years on admission, all cases who met the following criteria were identified: (i) first episode reported in the medical notes between 1977 and 1985, (ii) had neurological abnormalities on examination, (iii) were thought by a neurologist to have probable or definite MS, (iv) had a minimum of a further two out of the remaining four diagnostic criteria recommended by Schumacher,[9] (v) were white, (vi) were currently living in Leicestershire, and (vii) had approval from the general practitioner (GP) to be approached.

The GP for each case was traced by the Leicestershire Family Health Services Authority register. A bank of four female controls, who were within 2.5 years either side of the age of each case, were randomly selected from the same GP list. GPs were contacted to obtain their approval to approach the patient and for information about the patient's condition and knowledge of the diagnosis. Controls were excluded if they were reported by their GP as having neurological disorders or if they were not white.

3   Cases and controls received a full dental examination performed by an experienced dentist at home. Information on the presence, integrity and type of filling of every tooth surface was collected and recorded on a standard dental grid. The decayed, missing and filled index of dental caries for teeth (DMFT) was calculated for each person.[10] The number of teeth restored with amalgam, non-amalgam, either form of filling and crowns was also identified. The number of crowns were not included in the calculation of the DMFT because no information was available for the reason the crown was placed. Recent dental hygiene was estimated on the basis of current dental cleanliness assessed on a defined 3-point scale as 'good', 'fair' or 'poor'. Longer term dental hygiene was estimated on the basis of gingival health on a similar 3-point scale.[11] Enquiry was also made of any difficulty experienced with cleaning teeth and the frequency of attending a dentist.

4   Cases and controls were visited by a physician to obtain a blood sample and provide instruction on collecting a urine sample. The urinary mercury: creatinine ratio (nmol per mol) was measured using the method of cold vapour atomic absorption spectrophotometry.[12] Early morning midstream urine samples were collected in acid-washed glass beakers to minimise problems of contamination. Blood lead was determined using electrothermal atomisation atomic absorption spectrometry following venepuncture using steret and wipe.[13] Subsequently, blood mercury was determined, using stored blood, to eliminate any possibility of conversion or other means of elevation of organic mercury levels.[14]

5   Background information on cases and controls was obtained for a range of social and economic indicators. The levels of educational qualification achieved was used to adjust for social differences prior to the onset of the disease. Educational qualification level correlates well with socio-economic group (Spearman's coefficient = 0.393, P-value < 0.001 on 7,790 subjects, as calculated using data from the General Household Survey).[15]

6   Statistical analysis was performed using conditional logistic regression with SAS statistical software. This enabled an estimate of the relative risk (odds ratio) for a risk variable to be obtained. This relative risk is the multiplicative factor by which the odds of being a case is multiplied when the risk variable is increased by one unit. (If the risk factor is a 2-level dichotomous categorical variable and the first category is being compared with the second then it is assumed that the value of the first category is one unit larger than the second category). A 95% confidence interval (CI) for the relative risk and the p-value for the test of the null hypothesis that the odds ratio is unity were calculated.

Detecting disease 7

This chapter describes how to assess the efficacy of tests that detect disease. In dentistry, as in medicine, tests can be categorised into **diagnostic** tests or **screening** tests, and this is a useful distinction.

The purpose of a diagnostic test is to identify with almost complete certainty whether an individual has a disease or not. Such tests are effective in identifying disease but they can be expensive and/or harmful to the individual. A screening test cannot identify people with and without disease with certainty. It will always miss some people with the disease and it will always incorrectly classify some people as having the disease when they do not. The purpose of a screening test is to identify people who are at a **high risk** of having a disorder now (which can be confirmed by a diagnostic test) or people who are at high risk of acquiring the disorder in the future. Screening tests are usually harmless and/or relatively cheap. When a diagnostic test is not available a screening test is useful because it can identify those who are at a high risk so that these people can be given some preventive treatment.

Screening is the identification of asymptomatic people who are at a high risk of having or developing disease, and who can benefit from further investigation and treatment, or some preventive strategy. For a screening programme to be considered worthwhile, there are several requirements that should be fulfilled[1] (Box 7.1). This chapter is based around the published paper reproduced on pp. 165–171 and each of these requirements will be discussed in relation to the paper.

Reference: Downer, M.C., Evans, A.W., Hughes Hallett, C.M., Jullien, J.A., Speight, P.M. and Zakrzewska, J.M. Evaluation of screening for oral cancer and precancer in a company headquarters. *Comm Dent Oral Epidemiol* 1995;**23**:84–88.

Although the focus of this chapter is on assessing the effectiveness of a screening programme, some of the principles can also be applied to other types of test used to detect oral disease.

A screening programme aims either to identify people with disease and treat them successfully, or to identify those at high risk and prevent them from getting the disease

---

[1] Based on those by Wilson and Jungner 1968.

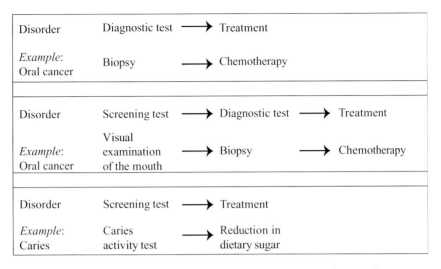

Figure 7.1 Different approaches to screening and diagnostic tests (with examples).

in the first place. Figure 7.1 illustrates three different ways in which diagnostic and screening tests can be used.

What is the aim of the study?

The aim is to identify oral cancer or precancerous lesions. The people included in the study worked in a single company, and they had not sought dental advice for cancer or precancer, and were therefore asymptomatic.

Box 7.1

Requirements for a worthwhile screening programme

1	Disorder	Needs to be well defined and medically important
2	Treatment	There should be an effective treatment or preventive remedy
3	Prevalence or incidence	Needs to be known and judged to be sufficiently high
4	Test	It should be simple and safe, easily implemented and easily made widely available
5	Performance	The distributions of test values should be known in affected and unaffected people and there should be little overlap between them
6	Financial	The programme should be cost-effective
7	Access	Those who can benefit from screening should be able to have access to the programme
8	Ethical	The test and procedure(s) after a positive result should be acceptable to both the screener and the person screened

CONDITIONS FOR A WORTHWHILE SCREENING PROGRAMME

Disorder

Oral cancer is clearly an important medical disorder because, if left untreated, it can lead to death. Oral cancer and precancer are well defined. Oral cancer can be detected from biopsy and there are a number of clinically identifiable precursor lesions which constitute a detectable preclinical phase. In a screening programme we refer to people as being **affected** or **unaffected**: affected people are those who have the disease, unaffected people are those who do not*. In this study, an affected person is someone who has oral cancer or precancer, and an unaffected person is someone who does not. In this study, the screening test was followed by a diagnostic test performed by a specialist in oral medicine (*paragraph 8*) who undertook further investigations which included biopsy. The diagnostic test determined whether subjects were affected or unaffected. It is important that the diagnosis of the disease of interest is well defined and made according to accepted criteria. This is to ensure that all the affected people in the study have been diagnosed in a consistent way.

Treatment

Precancerous lesions can be managed by repeated clinical examinations. Oral cancer can be treated by surgery with or without radiotherapy. The earlier the diagnosis the better the chance of reduced morbidity and mortality.

Prevalence or incidence

Oral cancer is relatively rare in the UK, with about 4400 new cases per year, or an incidence rate of 7.5 per 100 000 per year[†]. Two-thirds are men and the risk increases with age. Smoking and alcohol drinking are established risk factors. The prevalence of oral cancer and precancer in this particular study can be obtained from Table 7.1 (taken from *Table 2* in the paper); of the 309 people who were screened, 17 were diagnosed as having cancer or precancer, representing a prevalence of 5.5%. Because of the clinical importance of oral cancer a prevalence of 5.5% may be judged sufficiently high to warrant a screening programme, if an effective test exists. Below, we discuss methods that can be used to describe the effectiveness of a screening test.

Test

The proposed screening test involves a visual examination of the mouth that is both simple and safe (*paragraph 6*). The test can be performed by any dentist and so is appropriate for general practice. After people have had a screening test they are classified as being either **screen-positive** or **screen-negative** (sometimes called **test-positive** and **test-negative**). If a person is classified as **screen-positive** they have been identified by the screening test as being at **high risk** of having the disorder; if classified as **screen-negative** the test identifies them as being **low risk**.

---

* Where the aim of screening is disease prevention, affected means those who will develop the disease over the next, say, 5 years and unaffected are those who will not.
[†] http://info.cancerresearchuk.org/cancerstats/oral/

Table 7.1 The number of people who were screen-positive and screen-negative according to whether they had oral cancer/precancer or not.

	Screening test result		
	Positive	**Negative**	
Definitive diagnosis			
Positive*	12 (a)	5 (b)	17
Negative	2 (c)	290 (d)	292
	14	295	309

* Has oral cancer or precancer.

We can illustrate how risk changes after screening by considering the results in Table 7.1. Before these people were screened their risk of oral cancer or precancer was 5.5%; the overall risk in this study. After screening, we have further information on people. If they are screen-positive their risk is now 86% (12/14) – increased from 5.5%. If they are screen-negative their risk is 1.7% (5/295) – decreased from 5.5%. It is important that the criteria for classifying people are clear and well defined. People in this particular study are classified as **screen-positive** if they had a white or red patch or an ulcer that had been present for 2 or more weeks. These lesions were then qualified based on the visual signs listed in *Table 1* in the paper. Box 7.2 summarises key points when thinking about the screening process.

Performance

There are two aspects of screening performance – the effectiveness of the test and what the test result means to the patient. A further aspect of screening is how well the test performs in a particular population.

Box 7.2

The screening process

We need to consider:	Example
What is the disorder?	Oral cancer or precancer
What is the screening test?	Visual inspection of the lips, mucosal surface of the mouth and oropharynx
What defines a person as screen-positive (high risk)?	White or red patch; ulcer present for ≥2 weeks
What happens to people who are screen-positive?	Examination by specialist, with biopsy if necessary

How good is the test at identifying people who have the disease and those who do not?

The performance of a test is measured by *both* the **detection rate** and **false-positive rate.** These can be obtained from a table of the type shown in Table 7.1 (*Table 2 of the paper*). Results from screening studies are often presented in this way.

The detection rate is the percentage of *affected* individuals who have *screen-positive* results (or the percentage of people who will develop the disease who are screen-positive). It measures how likely the test is to pick up someone if they have the disorder. The detection rate is sometimes called **sensitivity**. The higher the detection rate, the better the test. From Table 7.1, there are 17 people who were diagnosed as having cancer or precancer, and of these 12 were classified as test-positive by the screening test. The detection rate is therefore 71% (12 ÷ 17); 71% of people who have cancer or precancer are picked up by the test.

The false-positive rate is the percentage of *unaffected* individuals who have *screen-positive* results (or the percentage of people who will not develop the disease who are screen-positive). It measures how likely the test is to pick up someone if they do not have the disorder. A false-positive is someone identified as having a high risk of the disorder, but after further testing they are found to be disease free. When screening is aimed at prevention it is not possible to know for sure whether or not a person who is screen-positive will develop the disease, so if screen-positives receive treatment, there will also be some false-positives who would receive treatment unnecessarily. The lower the false-positive rate the better the test, because fewer unaffected people will be referred for further testing or treatment. In this study, the false-positives are people who do not have cancer or precancer but have been classified as positive by the screening test. From Table 7.1 there are 292 unaffected people, of whom 2 are classified as screen-positive by the screening test. The false-positive rate is thus 0.7% (2 ÷ 292); only 0.7% of people who do not have the disease are picked up as positive by

---

Box 7.3

	Screening test result	
	Positive	**Negative**
With disease	a	c
Without disease	b	d

$$\textbf{Detection rate} = \frac{a}{a+c} = \frac{\text{All those who are test-positive and have disease}}{\text{All with disease}}$$

$$\textbf{False-positive rate} = \frac{b}{b+d}$$

$$= \frac{\text{All those who are test-positive and do not have disease}}{\text{All without disease}}$$

the screening test. Box 7.3 shows how detection and false-positive rates are calculated in general.

Specificity is 100% − false-positive rate%. For the false-positive rate of 0.7% the specificity is 99.3%. The specificity is, therefore, the percentage of unaffected individuals who are classified correctly as being unaffected by the screening test. Although specificity is often used in the literature, the false-positive rate is of more practical use because these are the people who will have further testing and possibly unnecessary treatment even though they do not have the disease.

For this oral cancer screening test, the detection rate of 71% is high and the false-positive rate of 0.7% is low, indicating that the proposed test has a good chance of correctly identifying people with the disease and a low chance of saying that people have the disease when, in fact, they do not.

There are no 'ideal' values for the detection rate and false-positive rate. Whether a screening test is judged to be effective will depend on the particular disorder; its prevalence and severity, and what happens to screen-positives. For example, if a certain disorder is common and clinically important, a test that has a detection rate of 40% and a false-positive rate of 10% might be thought to be useful. Whereas if the disorder is rare, such a test would be judged to be ineffective because it would have a detection rate that is too low and a false-positive rate that is too high. The diagnostic tests or treatments that follow screening, and their possible harmful effects, should also be considered in relation to the number of false-positives. If these tests and treatments are cheap and relatively safe then a high false-positive rate may be acceptable. If the tests or treatments are potentially painful or harmful, it might be inappropriate to give them to too many unaffected people.

Once we have the detection rate and false-positive rate it is useful to look at their 95% confidence intervals. The detection rate and false-positive rate can only lie between 0% and 100%. The 95% confidence interval for the detection rate in this study is 46% to 96% (see footnote to *Table 2* in the paper). It is likely that the true effect of the test is that at least half of all people with cancer/precancer would be detected, but up to 96% could be identified. The 95% confidence interval for the false-positive rate is obtained by simply subtracting the 95% CI for the specificity from 100% (in the footnote to *Table 2*). It is 0% to 2%. This is a narrow range and the false-positive rate is low, indicating that the test is not picking up too many people who do not have the disease. Even if the most conservative estimates of the screening test from the confidence interval (detection rate = 46% and false-positive rate = 2%) were used the screening programme might still be considered worthwhile.

What does the test result mean to the patient?

What is important to the patient is the implication of the results for them. If the test result is positive, what is the chance that the patient has the disease? If the test is negative what is the chance that the patient does not have the disease? These are called, respectively, the **positive predictive value** (**PPV**) and the **negative predictive value** (**NPV**) of the test. Box 7.4 shows how these are calculated using the information in Table 7.1. The positive predictive value tells us that patients with a positive test

Box 7.4

How good is the screening test?	
How well does the test classify those with disease?	Detection rate DR = 12/17 = 71%
How well does the test classify those without disease?	False-positive rate FPR = 2/292 = 0.7%
What does the test result tell us?	
If the test is +ve what is the chance that the patient has the disease?	Positive predictive value PPV = 12/14 = 86%
If the test is −ve what is the chance that the patient does not have the disease?	Negative predictive value NPV = 290/295 = 98%

result have an 86% chance of having oral cancer or precancer. The negative predictive value tells us that patients with a negative test result have a 98% chance of not having oral cancer or precancer. Box 7.5 shows how positive predictive value and negative predictive value are calculated in general.

The screening test is only one part of a screening programme (it is followed by the diagnostic test, counselling and treatment options). How would the test will perform in *a given population*? This depends on how common the disease is (the prevalence or incidence). Table 7.2 shows how our test will work in the population of company employees in London where the prevalence of oral cancer and precancer was 5.5%.

Box 7.5

	Screening test result	
	Positive	**Negative**
With disease	a	c
Without disease	b	d

$$\text{Positive predictive value} = \frac{a}{a+b} = \frac{\text{All test-positive and with disease}}{\text{All test positive}}$$

$$\text{Negative predictive value} = \frac{d}{c+d} = \frac{\text{All test-negative and without disease}}{\text{All test negative}}$$

Table 7.2 Illustration of the outcome of a screening programme of 1000 people (prevalence of oral cancer and precancer is 5.5%).

		No. of people who are screen-positive	No. of people who have diagnostic test*	No. of people who receive treatment
No. of people to be screened	1000			
No. expected with disease (oral cancer)	55	43 (DR = 71%)	43	43
No. expected without disease	945	7 (FPR = 0.7%)	7	0
Positive predictive value			86% (43/50)	

* In this example we assume that all screen-positive patients had a diagnostic test but in other situations this may not be so.

We take a large number of people, say 1000, and we expect that among these there will be 55 with the disease and 945 without. The table shows what we expect would happen to this group of people as they go through the screening process.

If 1000 people are screened, 43 of the 55 affected individuals are expected to be screen-positive (detection rate = 43/55 = 71%), and 7 of the 945 unaffected individuals will be screen-positive (false-positive rate = 7/945 = 0.7%). At this stage, we would have 50 screen-positive people but we do not know for sure which have cancer or precancer and which do not. We then need to refer them all to a specialist (this is the diagnostic test) in order to identify those who have cancer or precancer. The positive predictive value tells us what proportion of the 50 screen-positive people who have been referred for diagnostic testing are expected to have cancer or precancer; here this is 43/50 = 86%.

These calculations assume that the diagnostic test has a detection rate of 100% (the specialist will correctly identify all of the people with cancer or precancer who are referred) and a false-positive rate of 0% (the specialist will not incorrectly diagnose a person as having cancer or precancer when they are unaffected). We have made this assumption to simplify the example. In practice, even diagnostic tests often have some small margin of error, for example the detection rate might be 98% rather than 100%.

Once we have laid out the results for a large screened population, as in Table 7.2, we can make a judgement over whether the screening programme is effective or not by describing its benefits and costs (Box 7.6). We consider whether the gain from implementing a screening programme is justified by the human costs (for example anxiety and any harm associated with the diagnostic test) and by the workload, including the financial costs (cost of the screening and diagnostic tests and of counselling people classified as screen-positive). In the screening programme in Table 7.2 we assume that all people who are screen-positive agreed to have the diagnostic test, and of those who had this test, all agreed to be treated. This is not often the case in practice, so the numbers would need to be adjusted to allow for people who refuse.

Box 7.6

Screening 1000 people

What has been gained?	What has screening involved?
43 people with oral cancer or precancer have been detected and treated	There have been: • 1000 oral examinations • 50 referred to oral specialist (diagnostic test) • 43 affected people treated for cancer/precancer • 7 unaffected people who would not have been seen by a specialist had they not been screened

In the example of oral cancer the study population came from a single company in London. There may be areas of the world where the disease is more common and areas where it is rare. What difference would this make to a screening programme? Because the detection rate and false-positive rate provide a measure of the performance of the test itself, they are not affected by the prevalence of the disorder and so should be similar across different populations. For example, the detection rate for the screening test in the study was 71%, so we should be able to detect 71% of whatever the number of affected people there are in a population, whether that be 71% of 10 or 71% of 1000. The positive predictive value, however, does depend on the particular population in which screening is to be conducted. If the prevalence changes so will the positive predictive value. Table 7.3 shows the results of a screening programme of 1000 people in the same way as in Table 7.2 but with a lower prevalence of oral cancer and precancer (2% instead of 5.5%).

The performance of the screening test is still the same as before. The detection and false-positive rates are practically the same in both examples, but the

Table 7.3 Illustration of the outcome of a screening programme of 1000 people (prevalence of oral cancer and precancer is 2%).

		No. of people who are screen-positive	No. of people who have diagnostic test*	No. of people who receive treatment
No. of people to be screened	1000			
No. expected with disease (oral cancer)	20	14 (DR = 70%)	14	14
No. expected without disease	980	7 (FPR = 0.7%)	7	0
Positive predictive value			67% (14/21)	

* In this example all screen-positive patients had a diagnostic test but in other situations this may not be so.

positive predictive value is now 67%, considerably worse than the positive predictive value of 86% when the prevalence was 5.5%. The positive predictive value decreases when the prevalence or detection rate decreases or the false-positive rate increases.

Financial

There will be several financial factors to consider, namely:

- *The cost of the screening test.* Because this is offered to everyone who may benefit from screening such costs usually need to be low.
- *The cost of the diagnostic test.* People who are screen-positive would be referred to a specialist who will diagnose whether they have oral cancer or precancer, or not. This examination(s) will be more expensive than the screening test, as it involves a variety of investigations which may include a biopsy.
- *The cost of treatment.* Once people with oral cancer and precancer have been identified they need to be offered treatment (for example surgery) or more intense follow-up.
- *The cost of any harm done.* Some diagnostic tests are associated with adverse effects, and there may be a financial cost associated with this. For example, in antenatal screening for Down's syndrome, the diagnostic test is an amniocentesis, which can cause miscarriage. In this screening programme for oral cancer and precancer there was no harm incurred by the diagnostic test.

Once these costs have been estimated, it is possible to calculate information such as:

- the total cost of screening 1000 people
- the cost of detecting one affected individual.

Access

Because the screening test is a visual inspection of the mouth, it can be performed by any dental practitioner, after sufficient training. Therefore, access to screening should be straightforward.

Ethical

Both the screening test and diagnostic test, and subsequent treatment should be acceptable to patients. Screening always causes anxiety; in this case, people who are classified as 'test positive' may feel alarmed by thinking that they might have cancer. Furthermore, among those who are given test-negative results, there will be some who have cancer or precancer (i.e. were missed by the screening test). The test result might offer false reassurance to these people.

Key points

- Screening on a large scale requires the disorder to be medically important with a prevalence (or incidence) that is sufficiently high.
- The performance of a screening or diagnostic test is quantified by the detection and false-positive rates.
- The performance of a test in a particular population is quantified by the positive predictive value and negative predictive value.
- Once people are diagnosed with disease, an effective treatment should be available.

Exercise

Consider the following questions in relation to the paper by Downer *et al.* (1995)

1. What was the screening uptake, i.e. the proportion of people approached who agreed to be screened?
2. There were no cases of carcinoma in the sample (*paragraph 14*). Why might this be expected?
3. What was the most common diagnosis among affected individuals?
4. In this study the positive predictive value was 86% (from Table 7.1). Express this as an odds (i.e. the ratio of the number with disease : number without disease, among those who are screen-positive) and interpret it.
5. Were the individuals screened in the study representative of all employees in the company? If not, would this affect screening performance?
6. Screening was undertaken by two dental practitioners (*paragraph 5*). What are an advantage and a disadvantage of only having two screeners in the study?
7. The two screeners in the study did not receive any specialist training (*paragraphs 5 and 17*). What effect might this have on (i) detection rate (ii) false-positive rate and (iii) positive predictive value?
8. What does the study contribute to dental practice?
9. If the prevalence of oral cancer or precancer was very low, say 1 in 10 000, would it be worthwhile to have a screening programme?

Answers on pp. 217–218

REFERENCE

1. Wilson J.M.G. and Jungner, G. *Principles and practice of screening for disease.* Public Health Papers No. 34. Geneva: World Health Organization, 1968.

Community Dent Oral Epidemiol 1995; 23: 84–8

**Community Dentistry
and Oral Epidemiology**

ISSN 0301-5661

Journal paper

Evaluation of screening for oral cancer and precancer in a company headquarters

**M.C. Downer[1],
A.W. Evans[1],
C.M. Hughes Hallett[2],
J.A. Jullen[1],
P.M. Speight[1] and
J.M. Zakrzewska[1]**

[1]Eastman Dental Institute,
[2]Unilever plc, London, UK

Downer MC, Evans AW, Hughes Hallett CM, Jullien JA, Speight PM, Zakrzewska JM: Evaluation of screening for oral cancer and precancer in a company headquarters. Community Dent Oral Epidemiol 1995; 23: 84–8. © Munksgaard, 1995

Abstract – Oral cancer and precancer appear to fulfil many of the criteria for a disease suitable for mass screening. Several commercial organisations in the UK have introduced screening for their employees. One program has been formally evaluated over the course of 1 yr. Of 553 company headquarters staff aged ≥40 yr, 292 (53%) responded to the well-publicised screening invitation and received a simple clinical examination of the oral mucosa from one of two company dentists. In addition, 17 staff were screened from a separate company worksite. After screening, subjects were examined independently by an oral medicine specialist with access to the relevant diagnostic aids. The dentists' screening decisions were validated against the specialist's definitive diagnoses (the 'gold standard'). The true prevalence of subjects with lesions diagnosed as positive (white patch, red patch or ulcer of greater than 2 weeks' duration) was 17 (5.5%). Overall, sensitivity was 0.71 and specificity, 0.99. The compliance rate to screening among headquarters subjects in seven occupational categories did not differ significantly from the occupational profile for all headquarters personnel. Estimates of relative risk of a positive diagnosis were calculated by logistic regression for five independent variables; gender, age, moderate smoking, heavy smoking, and smoking combined with greater than low risk alcohol consumption. Only heavy smoking (≥20 cigarettes per day) produced a significant odds ratio (3.43, $p < 0.05$).

Key words: compliance; oral cancer; oral precancer; relative risk; screening; sensitivity; specificity

M. C. Downer, Department of Dental Health Policy, Eastman Dental Institute, 256 Gray's Inn Road, London WC1X 8LD, United Kingdom

Accepted for publication
24 January 1994

1   There are some 2000 new cases of oral cancer reported in England and Wales each year with an overall incidence of 4.5 per 100 000 per annum. Approximately 60% of patients die from their disease within 5 yr (1). In the industrialized world it is considered the eighth most common cancer, representing between 1 and 2% of total malignancies, and there is evidence that incidence and mortality are increasing (2). Although cancer often apparently arises de novo,

there are also a number of clinically identifiable precursor lesions which constitute a detectable preclinical phase (3). Pre-malignant lesions such as leukoplakia, and other conditions associated with a high risk may be present in up to 5% of the population over 40 yr of age (4–6).

Treatment of oral cancer, especially advanced lesions, is associated with significant physical and psychological morbidity whereas small lesions are relatively easy to detect and treat effectively. Poor survival is in part due to a failure to detect small lesions since over 60% of patients present with lesions over 2 cm in diameter, by which stage prognosis is significantly worsened (3, 7). Yet it is recognised that a simple clinical examination can detect asymptomatic disease and result in treatment being instituted early (8). It seems timely therefore to consider the feasibility of screening for oral cancer and precancer. A recent report (9) concluded that oral cancer met most of the criteria of WILSON & JUNGNER (10) for a disease suitable for screening but found insufficient evidence to recommend a national screening program without further research.

In India, where the incidence of oral cancer is high, large scale primary preventive programs aimed at reducing tobacco usage have been evaluated (11). However, few studies have attempted specifically to validate clinical screening for oral cancer and precancer. Nevertheless there is evidence that satisfactory sensitivity and specificity levels can be achieved both by dentists (12) and, in developing countries, by primary health care workers (13).

IKEDA and coworkers (12) conducted their screening among factory and office workers in Japan. The workplace offers an ideal opportunity for screening (14–16) and although a number of companies have now instituted oral cancer and precancer screening for their employees (17), there have been no formal evaluations of worksite oral screening programs in the United Kingdom. The purpose of this project was to establish the sensitivity and specificity of a screening test for the detection of oral cancer and precancer, and to evaluate a pilot screening program in a workplace environment.

Material and methods

The screening program – Screening was carried out in the London headquarters of a large commercial company. All staff aged 40 yr or over were invited to attend for an oral screening in the surgeries of the on-site company dental practice. The program was widely publicised through the company house magazine, a video screen in the entrance hallway, and by means of an information sheet explaining the importance of mouth screening in the detection of cancer and the nature of the examination.

Screening was conducted at dedicated sessions and was carried out by two general dental practitioners who had not received any specific training except for instruction in the screening procedure and the criteria for a positive or negative test.

The screening test consisted of a thorough, systematic visual examination of the lips and mucosal surface of the mouth and oropharynx. It was carried out under a dental operating light using two mouth mirrors to retract and visualise the soft tissues and a gauze swab to manipulate the tongue. The test was recorded as positive if a white patch, red patch or ulcer of greater than 2 weeks' duration was detected. However, these criteria were further qualified by defining lesions or conditions regarded as malignant or premalignant and therefore screened positive, and by indicating lesions which might have a similar appearance but should be regarded as negative (Table 1). An apparently normal mucosa was also classified as negative. Findings were entered on a simple report form. In addition, each subject screened was asked to complete a brief, confidential questionnaire designed to identify high risk lifestyle factors, notably smoking and alcohol consumption habits. Questions covered the amount and type of tobacco used and the duration of use, and the amount, frequency and type of alcoholic drink consumed.

Table 1 Specific lesions or conditions to be regarded as positive or negative in the screening program

Positive	Negative
carcinoma	geographic tongue
leukoplakia	median rhomboid glossitis
erythroplakia	pseudomembranous candidosis
lichen planus	aphthous ulceration
lupus erythematosus	transient white patches
submucous fibrosis	stomatitis nicotina
actinic keratosis	

7   The program was designed to continue long term, and a pathway was established for patients requiring referral. Also all participants were given preventive advice stressing the risk factors for oral cancer and the benefits of a healthy lifestyle.

8   *Evaluation and analysis* – After screening, each subject was independently examined by a specialist in oral medicine who was unaware of the findings of the screener but who had the subject's completed lifestyle questionnaire available for scrutiny. The reference criterion ("gold standard") for calculating sensi-tivity and specificity was the definitive diagnosis by the specialist who had access to any relevant diagnostic aids, including biopsy if considered necessary.

9   Sensitivity and specificity were computed for each screener separately and for their combined results. Uptake of the program among staff was recorded, and the classification of screened subjects by occupational group was compared for goodness-of-fit with the occupational profile of all eligible staff on the headquarters payroll. Seven occupational staff grades were used for classification purposes. Logistic multiple regression analysis estimating relative risk was carried out using the specialist definitive diagnosis, classified as negative or positive, as the dependent variable. Personal data items and responses from the lifestyle questionnaire, each aggregated and expressed in binary form, represented the independent risk factor variables. The variable, age, was entered as a continuous independent measurement. The cut-points for the dichotomized variables were (1) any use, (2) moderate or (3) heavy usage of tobacco, and (4) higher than safe use of alcohol. The criteria are specified in Table 5.

Results

There were 553 eligible staff aged 10 40 yr or over on the headquarters payroll and 292 (53%) were screened during the 1-year evaluation period. Seventeen staff were also screened from a separate worksite of the company and included in the analysis. Of those screened, all but 12 were registered patients of the practice.

Table 2 presents a contin- 11 gency table for frequencies of subjects classified as positive and negative according to the screening test and definitive diagnosis. Seventeen positive lesions were diagnosed by the specialist amounting to a prevalence of 5.5% in the screened population. There were five false-negative and two false-positive screening decisions, giving an overall sensitivity of 0.71 (95% CI, 0.46–0.96) and specificity of 0.99 (95% CI, 0.98–1.00). The positive predictive value of the screening test was 0.86. 12

Each screener saw only those subjects who presented for screening at their own scheduled sessions whereas the specialist was in attendance at every dedi-

Table 2 Contingency table of frequencies of positive and negative classifications of subjects according to screening test and definitive diagnosis, together with sensitivity and specificity values

		Test findings		True prevalence
		Positive	Negative	
Definitive diagnosis	Positive	12	5	17
	Negative	2	290	292
Test prevalence		14	295	309

Sensitivity = 0.71 (95% CI, 0.46–0.96), specificity = 0.99 (95% CI, 0.98–1.00).

Table 3 Comparison of uptake of the screening programme by headquarters staff according to occupational profile of all headquarters staff aged 40 yr or over

	Serv.	Cler.	Serv.	Asst. man.	Midd. man.	Sen. man.	Board memb.	All staff
All staff	57	57	62	93	154	119	11	553
% of total	10.3	10.3	11.2	16.8	27.8	21.5	2.0	100
Screened staff	17	33	30	65	85	57	5	292
Proportion of staff screened to total	0.30	0.60	0.48	0.74	0.60	0.50	0.45	0.56

Chi square $= 12.17$, 6 df, $P > 0.05$.

cated screening session and saw the screened subjects of both dentists. One screener returned a sensitivity of 0.75 (95% CI, 0.50–1.00) and the other, a value of 0.60 (95% CI, 0.17–1.00). Both had specificity values of 0.99 (95% CI, 0.98–1.00 and 0.97–1.00 respectively).

13   In Table 3, the composition of the headquarters group who presented themselves for screening according to occupational grade, is compared with the occupational profile of all eligible headquarters staff. The personnel department graded the staff as service (skilled and semi-skilled manual workers); clerical or secretarial; assistant, middle or senior management; and board members. The composition of the screened group by occupational grade did not differ significantly from that of all headquarters staff ($P > 0.05$). However, there was a trend towards an over-representation of assistant managers and an under-representation of service personnel.

Table 4 examines the subjects 14 who were diagnosed as positive according to their gender, age, occupational grading, and type of lesion diagnosed. There were nine cases of leukoplakia (2.9%), and eight cases of lichen planus (2.6%). There were no cases of squamous cell carcinoma. In establishing the definitive diagnosis, five patients were biopsied; two showed epithelial dysplasia, two hyper-keratosis without dysplasia and one, erosive lichen planus.

Table 5 presents the logistic 15 multiple regression analysis producing estimates of relative risk among those screened with five independent variables included. The only independent variable which was statistically significant ($P < 0.05$) was heavy smoking. This produced an odds ratio (estimating relative risk) of 3.43 (95% CI, 1.06–11.11) of a positive diagnosis for those who smoked 20 or more cigarettes or equivalent per day. The regression coefficients for the other independent variables

Table 4 List of subjects diagnosed as positive with gender, age (in years), occupational group, and diagnosed lesion

No.	M/F	Age	Occupation group	Diagnosed lesion
1	F	52	Middle manager	Erosive lichen planus
2	M	57	Service staff	Leukoplakia
3	M	47	Middle manager	Reticular lichen planus
4	M	55	Middle manager	Leukoplakia
5	M	61	Service staff	Reticular lichen planus
6	F	45	Assistant manager	Leukoplakia
7	F	57	Clerical staff	Reticular lichen planus
8	M	56	Senior manager	Leukoplakia
9	M	53	Senior manager	Leukoplakia
10	M	42	Middle manager	Leukoplakia
11	F	42	Middle manager	Erosive lichen planus
12	M	55	Assistant manager	Reticular lichen planus
13	M	48	Service staff	Leukoplakia
14	F	55	Assistant manager	Reticular lichen planus
15	M	55	Senior manager	Leukoplakia
16	M	54	Senior manager	Atrophic lichen planus
17	F	41	Middle manager	Leukoplakia

Journal paper

were non-significant ($P > 0.05$). In testing for goodness-of-fit of the model, the chi-square value for -2 log likelihood with all conditions included was 124.35 ($P = 1.00$) and for goodness-of-fit, 292.13 ($P > 0.50$), upholding the null hypothesis that the model did not differ significantly from a "perfect" model.

Discussion

16 The response rate over the course of 1 yr to the offer of mouth screening for oral cancer and associated precancerous lesions amounted to 53% of all headquarters staff of 40 years of age or over. This appears rather low compared, for example, with the workplace screening program of IKEDA *et al.* (18), who recorded attendance rates of 77% and 60% in factory and office workers from 2 Japanese companies. However, the present figure represents some under-estimation of true compliance. A number of staff who were screened will not have been included in the evaluation since they were unable to attend at one of the dedicated sessions and were therefore not examined by the specialist diagnostician. The lower compliance rate in the present study rnay be due to the nature of the publicity material given to staff which was fairly forthright in its emphasis of the dangers of oral cancer, and uncompromising in its reference to the risk factors. A higher compliance might have been achieved with a more bland invitation to undergo general mouth, as opposed to oral cancer, screening. This would place a positive emphasis on the benefits of a healthy mouth rather than following a more negative approach centered on the detection of disease.

The overall sensitivity of the 17 screening test in the hands of the two company dentists amounted to 0.71 and compares with the value of 0.48 reported by IKEDA *et al.* (12) and 0.95 reported by WARNAKULASURIYA & PINDBORG (13) in their Sri Lanka study using primary health care workers. Two factors may have accounted for the comparatively low sensitivity achieved in the current study. First, there was no specific training and standardization of the screeners nor assessment of their performance before commencement. They were simply given the criteria for a positive or negative screen (Table 1) and instructed on the conduct of the evaluation and how to complete the recording forms. This was done purposely to test the ability of dental practitioners without special training to screen for oral cancer and

Table 5 Logistic multiple regression analysis with definitive diagnosis as dependent variable and gender, age and reported life style factors as independent variables

Independent variable	b coefficient (SE)	P	Odds ratio	95% confidence interval for OR
Gender	0.21 (0.53)	>0.05	1.23	0.43–3.51
Age (yr)	0.03 (0.04)	>0.05	1.03	0.95–1.11
Moderate smoker	−0.39 (0.79)	>0.05	0.68	0.14–3.21
Heavy smoker	1.23 (0.60)	>0.05	3.43	1.06–11.11
Drinker	−6.09 (37.55)	>0.05	0.00	2.48×10^{-35}–2.07×10^{29}
Smoker & drinker	−0.84 (46.68)	>0.05	0.43	7.91×10^{-41}–2.35×10^{39}
Constant	−4.72 (2.22)	>0.05	—	—

Key		
Variable	Specification	
Gender	Male = 1, female = 0	
Smoker	Current smoker of tobacco in any form or regular smoker within last 10 yr = 1, non-smoker (currently or for at least 10 yr) = 0	
Moderate smoker	Current smoker of less than 20 cigarettes or equivalent per day = 1, non-smoker = 0	
Heavy smoker	Current smoker of 20 or more cigarettes or equivalent per day = 1, non-smoker = 0	
Drinker	Consumer of more than 21 standard units of alcohol (male) or 14 units (female) per week = 1, drinker of less than the specified amount = 0	

precancer. Secondly, 96% of those screened were registered patients of the practice and the two practitioners were therefore aware that the patients were under continuing supervision. This may have made them cautious in designating a patient as positive. It is evident that thorough training in oral soft tissue screening is essential for those involved in any substantive program.

[18]   In contrast to sensitivity, specificity values were very high. There was thus a low to negligible frequency of false-positive decision making which is of some psychological importance to those screened and potential economic importance to providers of follow-up secondary care services (19). Of the five false-negative screening decisions, 3 were reticular lichen planus. Only two cases, apparently missed, were potentially serious conditions, one of erosive lichen planus and one of leukoplakia.

[19]   The occupational profile of the reened subjects did not differ significantly from that of the eligible headquarters population. Nevertheless, there was a degree of over-representation of the lower management grade and under-representation of service personnel. This reflects the pattern of uptake of oral care services generally where it is found that people in the professional and managerial social classes consistently have the higher asymptomatic attendance rates. Special efforts should be made in work-site screening programs for oral cancer to encourage staff in lower occupational grades to participate since some may be at heightened risk to the disease (20).

[20]   The logistic regression analysis, estimating the relative risk of having a positive lesion, incorporated five independent variables concerned with known risk factors. The cut-points were derived from a consideration of documents responding to government targets for reducing dependency on smoking and alcohol (21, 22). It produced a significant regression coefficient only in those claiming to smoke 20 or more cigarettes per day who had an estimated risk more than three times greater than non-smokers. However, the numbers involved in the analysis were small and quantification of the independent variables depended upon self-reported behaviour, which may be a doubtful reflection of actual behaviour.

[21]   The study has highlighted some of the difficulties of conducting a rigorous research program in a real life setting. Ideally, all those involved in data collection in a field research study should be unfamiliar with the subjects of the investigation. A larger study among dental hospital patients and subjects recruited from a medical practice list, currently being undertaken by the investigative team, should overcome this shortcoming. Despite the relatively small numbers, a quantifiable risk from heavy smoking was detected. Also a need was identified for specific training in the theory and practice of screening in order to maximise sensitivity while at the same time maintaining a low false-positive rate.

[22]   In conclusion, the study afforded a pragmatic evaluation of a screening program which is already established, and provided a useful pilot exercise for gaining practical experience and expertise in further investigations of the feasibility, suitability, and cost effectiveness of screening for oral cancer and precancer.

Acknowledgement – The authors are grateful to Ms AVIVA PETRIE for her valuable advice on the statistical analysis.

References

1. HINDLE I, NALLY F. Oral cancer: a comparative study between 1962–67 and 1980–84 in England and Wales. *Br Dem J* 1991; *170*: 15–9.

2. JOHNSON NW, WARNAKULA-SURIYA KAAS. Epidemiology and aetiology of oral cancer in the United Kingdom. *Community Dent Health* 1993; *10* (Suppl. 1): 13–29.

3. SPEIGHT PM, MORGAN PR. The natural history and pathology of oral cancer and precancer. *Community Dent Health* 1993; *10* (Suppl. 1): 31–41.

4. BANOCZY J, RIGO O. Prevalence study of oral precancerous lesions within a complex screening system in Hungary. *Community Dent Oral Epidemiol* 1991; *19*: 265–7.

5. BOUQUOT JE, GORLIN RJ. Leukoplakia, lichen planus, and other oral keraloses in 23,616 white Americans over the age of 35 years. *Oral Surg Oral Med Oral Pathol* 1986; *61:* 373–81.

6. KLEINMAN DV, SWANGO PA, NIESSEN LC. Epidemiologic studies of oral mucosal conditions – methodologic issues. *Community Dent Oral Epidemiol* 1991; *19:* 129–40.

7. PLATZ H, FRIES R, HUDEC M. eds. *Prognosis of oral cavity carcinomas. Results of a multicentric retrospective observational study.* Munich: Hanser, 1986.

8. ZAKRZEWSKA JM, HINDLE I, SPEIGHT PM. Practical considerations for the establishment of an oral cancer screening programme. *Community Dent Health* 1993; *10* (Suppl. 1): 79–85.

9. SPEIGHT PM, DOWNER MC, ZAKRZEWSKA J. eds. Screening for oral cancer and precancer report of a UK working group. *Community Dent Health* 1993; *10* (Suppl. 1): 1–89.

10. WILSON JMG, JUNGNER G. Principles and practice of screening for disease. Public Health

Papers. No. 34. Geneva: World Health Organization, 1968.

11. GUPTA PC, MEHTA FS, PINDBORG JJ, BHONSLE RB, MURTI PR, DAFTARY DK, AGHI MB. Primary prevention trial of oral cancer in India: a 10-year follow-up study. *J Oral Pathol Med* 1992; *21:* 433–9.

12. IKEDA N, ISHII T, IIDA S, KAWAI T. Mass screening for oral cancer and precancer in Japan. The first Asia-Pacific Workshop for Oral Mucosal Lesions. Abstract 1–6, 1992.

13. WARNAKULASURIYA S, PINDBORG JJ. Reliability of oral precancer screening by primary health care workers in Sri Lanka. *Community Dent Health* 1990; *7:* 73–9.

14. RATCLIFFE JM, HALPERIN WE, FRAZIER TM, SUNDIN DS, DELANEY L, HORNUNG RW. The prevalence of screening in industry: report from the National Institute for Occupational Safety and Health National Occupational Hazard Survey. *J Occupational Med* 1986; *28:* 906–12.

15. THORNTON J, CHAMBERLAIN J. Crevical screening in the workplace. *J Community Med* 1989; *11:* 290–8.

16. RASMUSSEN K, LUNOE-JENSON P, SVANE O. Biological monitoring and medical screening at the workplace in the EC countries. *Int Arch Occupational Environmental Health* 1991; *63:* 347–52.

17. FEAVER GP. Screening for oral cancer and precancer. *Dent Practice* 1990; *28:* 14–8.

18. IKEDA N, ISHII T, IIDA S, KAWAI T. Epidemiological study of oral leukoplakia based on mass screening for oral mucosal diseases in a selected Japanese population. *Community Dent Oral Epidemiol* 1991; *19:* 160–3.

19. CHAMBERLAIN J. Evaluation of screening for cancer. *Community Dent Health* 1993; *10* (Suppl. 1): 5–11.

20. BLINKHORN AS, JONES JH. Behavioural aspects of oral cancer screening. *Community Dent Health* 1993; *10* (Suppl. 1): 63–9.

21. CHAMBERS J, KILLORAN A, MCNEILL A, REID D. The Health of the Nation: responses. Smoking. *Br Med J* 1991; *303:* 973–7.

22. ANDERSON P. The Health of the Nation: responses. Alcohol as a key area. *Br Med J* 1991; *303:* 766–9.

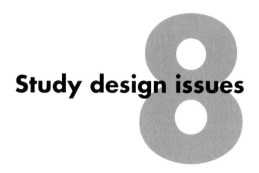

Study design issues

In the previous chapters we looked at a variety of study designs and statistical analyses in a selection of published papers. In this chapter we describe what sort of contribution different types of study make to the evidence base for dentistry and discuss some important aspects of study design.

TYPES OF STUDY

When we do research on people we have two possibilities: we can perform an experiment or we can observe what is happening without intervening. In some studies we may simply be interested in describing the prevalence of disease or other characteristics of the study population. In other studies we look for associations between disease and some other factor, either a risk factor or a treatment.

Clinical trials are used to examine the efficacy of treatments and preventive regimens, while observational studies are usually used to identify risk factors and causes of disease. In these studies we investigate the effect of an **exposure** or **treatment** on an **outcome** (Box 8.1). All studies on people are governed by ethical considerations. Although, theoretically, it would be possible to investigate the effect of risk factors for disease using clinical trials, in practice we do not conduct experiments that would intentionally result in some people suffering harm. In clinical trials, it is only ethical to randomise people to different treatments if we are not sure which one will be most effective. Before subjects consent to enter any study, there is an ethical obligation to provide them with sufficient information about the study, its aims and what will happen to the participants. Obtaining patient consent is a legal requirement in a clinical trial.

SELECTING THE SAMPLE

The way we select samples of people is different in observational studies and clinical trials. In observational studies a large group of people is identified and some are selected to be in our sample, using a method called **random sampling**. In clinical trials people who fulfil the selection criteria are invited to participate in the trial, and if they

Box 8.1

	Type of study		Exposure or treatment		Outcome
Experimental	Clinical trial	to investigate the effect of	Acupuncture	on	Pain
	Clinical trial	to investigate the effect of	Sedative gases	on	Successfully completing treatment
Observational	Cohort study	to investigate the effect of	Smoking	on	Periodontitis
	Case–control study	to investigate the effect of	Amalgam fillings	on	Multiple sclerosis
	Cross-sectional study	to investigate the association between	Year of study	and	Alcohol use

agree they are allocated to receive one of the trial treatments using randomisation, this is called **random allocation**.

To undertake **random sampling** we need a list of people who are representative of the population of interest, a **sampling frame**, from which to choose the sample. Examples of these might be all the patients aged under 16 years on the list of a dental practice, all the patients attending outpatients at a dental hospital over 1 year, or all the patients with multiple sclerosis identified from all the hospitals in one health authority. A **simple random sample** is one in which every individual in the sampling frame has an equal chance of being included in the sample.

For **random allocation** we first define a **target population** using inclusion and exclusion criteria. When patients fulfilling all of the criteria present for treatment they are then randomized to one of the trial treatments. For example, in the trial on acupuncture (see Chapter 5), some of the inclusion criteria were that patients were aged 18–40 years, in good health and eligible for extraction of an implanted third molar; an exclusion criterion was history of prior treatment with acupuncture. Patients who agreed to participate were then allocated to a treatment using randomisation. In **simple randomisation** every individual has an equal chance of being allocated to a particular treatment, and this should mean that any patient characteristic that might affect outcome will be distributed fairly evenly across the different treatments.

SAMPLE SIZE

A crucial aspect of study design is deciding how many subjects to include. If the study is too small then we may miss clinically important differences. If it is too

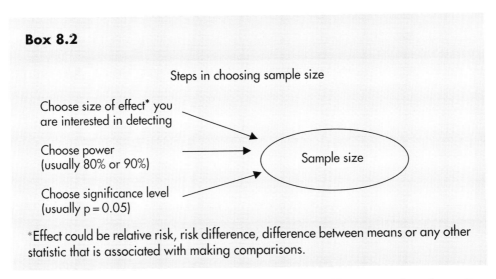

Box 8.2

Steps in choosing sample size

Choose size of effect* you
are interested in detecting

Choose power
(usually 80% or 90%)

Sample size

Choose significance level
(usually p = 0.05)

*Effect could be relative risk, risk difference, difference between means or any other statistic that is associated with making comparisons.

large, we waste resources and delay decisions that could improve dental practice. When making comparisons between groups there are formal statistical techniques for estimating sample size that ensure that if a clinically important effect does exist the study should be large enough to detect it. The calculation of sample size always requires that we specify three things: expected size of the effect (difference) that we are investigating; significance level; and power (Box 8.2).

Expected size of the effect

In order to decide on a sample size we need to have some idea of the size of difference we are looking for. It may seem counterintuitive to try to guess what the results of a study could be before we undertake it, but this process helps us to avoid doing studies that are much too large or too small to address the question of interest. For example, if we were investigating a new treatment for oral cancer, which is expected reduce five-year mortality by 10%, this would require a study involving several hundred people. If we did a much smaller study, of say 100 people, we would only be able to detect unrealistically large differences in mortality (say 50%). The effect could be expressed as a relative risk, risk difference, difference between means or some other statistic that is associated with making comparisons. The effect size that we choose to base our sample size on is often based on previous knowledge (from earlier research or observation). In the absence of such knowledge, the specified effect size may be the least that would be judged to be clinically important.

Significance level

At the end of the study we will perform a significance test and obtain a p-value. This will tell us how likely it is that an effect as large as the one we observe could have occured by chance. The p-value is the probability of making the erroneous conclusion that an effect exists when in fact there is no real effect. We would like this probability to be fairly small, and it is often set at 5%. Occasionally researchers want to be more certain that they will avoid this sort of error and specify a more stringent significance level, such as 1%.

Box 8.3

Example: Suppose our standard treatment has a cure rate of 75% and a new treatment is expected to have a cure rate of 90%

At the end of the trial we want to be able to say:
'A comparison of 90% vs 75% (i.e. a 15% difference) is statistically significant at the 5% level'

Power: We want an 80% probability of being able to make this statement. If there really is a difference of 15% or greater the power to detect such a difference will be 80%

Power

There are two ways in which we could draw the wrong conclusion about whether a difference or association exists. For simplification, throughout this discussion we will consider an effect size that is expressed as a difference between two groups, the concepts apply equally to measures of association. We could conclude that a difference exists, when, in fact, there is no real difference (as discussed in the preceeding paragraph). The other error we could make is to conclude that there is no difference, when, in fact a real difference does exist. To avoid this second type of error the study needs to be sufficiently large to detect a difference. **Power** is defined as the chance of detecting a specified difference (or effect size) if it really exists (Box 8.3). Power is usually set at 80% or 90%.

The aim of sample size estimation is to provide an *approximate* size for the study, that is, whether the study needs to have 100 patients or 500 – it does not matter if one sample size calculation gives 100 patients but another gives 110. There is always some guesswork involved in specifying the sample size, particularly in deciding on the effect size to use in the calculation, therefore estimates of study size are approximate and not precise.

The smaller the effect size the larger the study needs to be (Box 8.4). This is because it becomes more difficult to distinguish between a real difference and random variation. Suppose the effect of interest is the difference between the percentages of children completing dental treatment under two different anaesthetics. If we expect one anaesthetic to have a much larger effect than the other we would only need a small sample to show this. If we only expect a small difference between anaesthetics then we would need a large sample to detect this small difference.

Table 8.1 illustrates how sample size changes when the effect size or power changes, (it is based on the trial on sedative gases in Chapter 5). The significance level is set at 5%. We assume throughout that if given air, 50% of children would complete dental surgery. We then need to make a realistic guess at how many children might complete surgery if they were given sedative gas. If we think the effect size is likely to be small,

Box 8.4

Sample size goes up:

as effect size (difference) goes down	$\longrightarrow$	harder to detect small differences than big ones
as power goes up	$\longrightarrow$	increases the chance of picking up a difference
as significance level goes down	$\longrightarrow$	decreases the chance of saying there is a difference when there really is not

for example, a difference of only 10%, we would need a trial of 776 children, to achieve 80% power. This means that if sedative gas really does increase the completion rate to 60%, when we do the trial we will have an 80% chance of finding a significant difference at the 5% level (i.e. the p-value for the comparison of 50% versus 60% will be ≤0.05). For the same power, if we think the sedative gas is likely to have a very large effect, say a difference of 40%, we would need a trial of only 40 children. If we do a trial of only 40 children then we may miss any real effect that is less than 40%, so even if we find a difference of 20%, our sample size will be too small for us to be able to say that this is a statistically significant difference.

Sample size is a fundamental issue when considering research results. If a study is much larger than it needs to be to answer the research question, then we waste resources, and, in the case of clinical trials, may be giving some people an inferior treatment unnecessarily. However, an over-large study will give us a clear answer to the research question. Resources might be saved by doing a small study, but we may miss a clinically important difference because we find no statistically significant difference between two treatments, when in fact there is a real difference: our study is just too small to detect it. So what can we infer when a difference (say between two treatments) is reported to be 'not statistically significant'? There are three possible explanations for such a finding:

Table 8.1   The number of children needed in a trial comparing the effect of sedative gas versus air on the ability to complete dental treatment, according to effect size and power.

% expected to complete treatment with		Effect size	Power		
Gas	Air	Difference (Gas – Air)	80%	85%	90%
60%	50%	10%	776	886	1038
70%	50%	20%	186	214	250
80%	50%	30%	78	88	104
90%	50%	40%	40	44	52

* all sample sizes are based on a 5% significance level

- There really is no difference.
- There is a difference, but by chance we picked a sample that did not show this.
- There is a difference but the study had **insufficient power** to detect it; the study was too small.

We cannot conclude that the two treatments have an equivalent effect, this is only one *possible* explanation for the non-significant result. The crucial alternative explanation is that there could be a real underlying difference, but because the study was too small it did not have the power to show this. Whatever the measure of effect used in a study, relative risk, risk difference, difference between two means, or regression or correlation coefficient, if the result is 'not statistically significant' it is important to be aware that there could still be a real and clinically important effect, but the study may have been too small to detect this.

MORE ON OBSERVATIONAL STUDIES

Cross-sectional studies are usually the quickest, simplest and cheapest type of study to do. We take a sample of people and record information about them at one point in time. Cross-sectional studies do not involve either the long follow-up of cohort studies or the gathering of retrospective information of case–control studies. The limitation of cross-sectional studies is that they tell us little about what is happening over time, and associations between risk factors with disease should be interpreted with caution. Looking at one point in time could mean that a survey is preferentially including people with long-term disease. This is illustrated in Figure 8.1, where a cross-sectional study would provide a snapshot at one point in time (say year 1996). Patient numbers 2 and 5 have the disease for only a short time and are therefore missed from the study.

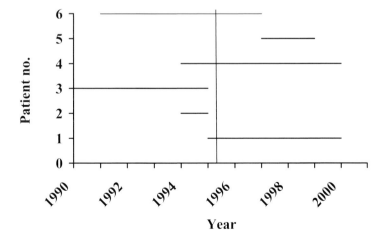

Figure 8.1 Hypothetical example illustrating the length of time that people have a disease. For example, patient 2 has the disease for a shorter duration than patient 4. The cross-sectional study is conducted in 1996. Each horizontal line represents the time during which a patient has the disease.

Box 8.5

	Cohort studies	**Case–control**
Length	Take a long time to do	Take a short time to do
Size	Large	Comparatively small
Cost	Expensive	Comparatively cheap
Outcome	Unsuitable for rare outcomes	Can be used for rare outcomes
Exposure	Collected prospectively	Collected retrospectively
Biases	Subjects enter study before onset of disease: avoids recall bias	Subjects enter study with disease
	Prospective exposure data: less recall bias	Retrospective exposure data: may introduce recall bias
	Easier to find subjects without disease; they come from the same population as subjects with disease	Sometimes difficult to find suitable controls (subjects without the disease), choice of control may introduce selection bias

Suppose we survey people with gingivitis. The longer someone has the disease the more likely they are to be in our survey, so if we look for risk factors we are likely to find those associated with having long-term gingivitis, and these may be different from those associated with short-term gingivitis. Our sample may not be representative of the whole population of people with gingivitis.

Comparison of cohort and case control studies

Cohort and case–control studies provide us with tools for investigating risk factors for disease. Cohort studies are less prone to bias than case–control studies for two reasons. First, they have the advantage of starting before the onset of disease and exposure, thus avoiding recall bias. Second, in case–control studies it can be difficult to decide on a control group because sometimes the choice of controls can lead to selection bias. A disadvantage of cohort studies is that they can take many years to do, because a sufficient number of people in the cohort have to develop disease. Cohort studies are not often used for looking at rare diseases, because the sample size would have to be prohibitively large. Box 8.5 summarises some of the main strengths and limitations of cohort and case–control studies.

In all studies we want the groups with and without disease to be as similar as possible except for the exposure, this is to minimise the possibility of bias and confounding.

BIAS

Bias is any systematic influence which results in an estimate from a study that tends to overestimate or underestimate the true (population) value. Bias can arise either from the way a study is designed or from the way it is conducted. Unlike confounding, which can be allowed for in the statistical analysis, there is usually little that can be done about bias. If, for example, in a case–control study we compare levels of smoking between cases with lung cancer and controls who were hospitalised for other respiratory diseases, we will underestimate the true effect of smoking on lung cancer, because smoking is also associated with other lung diseases. No statistical analysis can adjust for this adequately.

Biases arise from two main sources, subjects or errors of measurement. If the subjects we have chosen to be in the study are inherently different in some way between the comparison groups then any comparison will be affected. If the measurement of the risk factor of interest is influenced by the fact that people belong to one comparison group or another this will also distort our conclusions. For example, if people with high alcohol intake tend to under-report their consumption then, in the study exploring the association between alcohol and periodontitis, we might underestimate the strength of the association.

Biases that arise from the way the sample is chosen or recruited

Selection or allocation bias. Selection bias arises when the sample of participants in the study are chosen in such a way that some or all of them have characteristics that are not representative of the population of interest. This can happen when there is preferential selection of the subjects that is related to their case/control status or exposure status. Allocation bias can occur in clinical trials if certain types of patients (for example, with severe disease) are more likely to be given the active treatment. The sort of bias that is likely to arise depends, in part, on the study design. Examples of selection or allocation bias are:

- In a cross-sectional study of periodontitis done at one point in time there may be an excess of people with long-term disease
- In a case–control study of oral cancer and alcohol, if both cases and controls were identified from hospital patients, the controls might not be representative of the general population (they may be more likely to have alcohol-related illnesses).
- In a clinical trial, allocation bias occurs when patients who are likely to have a worse outcome are allocated to a particular treatment (this can be avoided by using randomisation).

Response bias. People who agreed to participate in the study (**responders**) are different from those who do not (**non-responders**). An example of response bias could be in a study of oral hygiene, where patients who practise good oral hygiene might be more likely to respond than patients with poor oral hygiene.

Biases associated with measurement of exposure or disease
From patients:

- *Recall bias*. Patients with disease may recall past experiences differently from patients without disease. This is particularly a problem in case–control studies where exposure data are retrospective. For example, in a case–control study of oral cancer, cases may be more likely to report past smoking accurately than controls.

- *Withdrawal bias*. Patients who withdraw from a study are likely to differ from those who do not. If withdrawal rates differ between the exposed and unexposed subjects this can create bias. In a clinical trial it is not uncommon for more patients on one treatment to withdraw from the trial than patients on the other treatment, particularly if the treatment is harder to tolerate. For example, patients having intensive chemotherapy may be more likely to withdraw from treatment than patients having surgery.
- *Follow-up bias*. The reason for lack of follow-up relates to exposure and differs between groups. For example, in a cohort study looking at the effect of smoking on the risk of developing periodontitis, heavy smokers may be more likely than never-smokers to be lost to follow-up because of smoking related illnesses.

From researchers:

- *Assessment bias*. If the clinician or patient is aware of the treatment allocated they may rate the results on the new treatment better than on the old. For example, a patient suffering chronic pain might be inclined to believe that a new treatment will have more effect than a treatment that they have tried before.
- *Interviewer bias*. If the interviewer is aware of the patient's disease status this may influence the way they conduct the interview. In a study of the association between smoking and periodontitis, the interviewer might ask more questions about the smoking habits of a subject known to have periodontitis.

Another bias can arise if a study involves asking about other specific medical conditions. People with the disease of interest may have undergone a range of diagnostic tests, which means that they are more likely to know if they have other diseases than people without the disease who have not been through the same battery of tests.

Clinical trials are less likely to suffer from bias than observational studies. Randomisation and blinding can be used to reduce or eliminate the possibility of allocation or assessment bias, and withdrawal bias is dealt with by intention-to-treat analysis. Case–control studies are prone to selection bias, through the choice of controls, and recall bias, because exposure data are collected retrospectively. Cohort studies avoid these biases because they start before the onset of disease, and people with and without disease come from the same population.

CONFOUNDING

When we find an association between an exposure and an outcome, we have to consider whether it is likely to be real or whether it may be due to some other factor, a confounder. A variable is a confounder if it is independently associated with both the outcome and the explanatory variable in a study. Confounding can make relations appear that do not really exist, and can mask some relationships that do exist.

The commonest confounding factors are age, sex, and time. Suppose we look at the number of DMFT in people of different ethnic origins in the UK, and we find that one ethnic group has fewer decayed or missing teeth. This may be because this group is much younger than the others. A comparison among people of a similar age could show that the proportion of people with tooth decay and loss are, in fact, similar in different ethnic groups. There are methods for reducing the effect of confounding that can be applied either at the design or analysis stage of a study.

Dealing with confounding at the design stage
Clinical trials
The objective of randomisation is to allocate patients so that we produce treatment arms that are as similar as possible with regard to characteristics other than treatment, and the only systematic difference between the two arms is the treatment given. Randomisation should mean that any differences in results observed at the end of the trial are due to the effect of the treatment and not to any other factors. In very large trials randomisation almost always produces a good balance of prognostic factors. In smaller trials it may be necessary to be even more careful in ensuring that a potential confounding factor is balanced between treatment groups. Some investigators choose a randomisation method that will ensure that the treatment groups are balanced with regard to factors that are known to be associated with the outcome measure such as age or severity of illness. The most commonly used methods that are used to address this are **stratification** and **minimisation**. When these are referred to in papers it means that the treatment groups are likely to be balanced for the factors specified.

Confounding in observational studies
Confounding is inherent in many observational studies because there is no strategy like randomisation that we can use to avoid it. In case–control studies the effect of known confounders can be reduced by using **matching** as part of the sample selection process. To do this, we take each case and try to identify a control (or several controls) that matches the characteristics of this case as closely as possible. Suppose we are doing a study on nutrition and oral health based in several dental practices. We know that both age and social class are related to nutrition and to oral health, so they are potential confounders. A case is identified from one dental practice then we look on that practice list for a control who was aged within say two years of the case. People on the same practice list are likely to be more similar in socio-economic background than people from other practice lists, so this could also eliminate some of the difference in socio-economic status between cases and controls.

Dealing with confounding at the analysis stage
The type of statistical analysis undertaken to deal with confounding is determined by the design of the study and the type of data involved. Clinical trials are largely unaffected by confounding, and so tend to need relatively simple analyses because randomisation creates groups in which the only difference is the treatment received. Any difference in outcome is likely to be due to the treatment, so this is usually all we need to consider in the analysis.

Observational studies require more complex analyses, because the exposure groups may differ on many other characteristics, so in the analysis we will have to tease out the effect of many different factors rather than just one. The statistical techniques used to do this are called **multiple logistic regression** and **multiple linear regression**. Which is appropriate depends on the type of outcome measured. Where the outcome is something we can count, like presence/absence of oral disease or dead/alive, logistic regression can be used. When the outcome involves taking measurements on people or objects, for example, optical density or blood pressure, linear regression is used. If a researcher uses methods like these in the statistical analysis, you know one or more confounders have been allowed for.

Interpretation of results from observational studies

Observational studies are more likely to be affected by bias and confounding, we therefore need to make a judgement on whether the size of the effect seen (for example, relative risk or odds ratio) might be greatly influenced by these factors. Would the relative risk become close to 1.0 (i.e. no association between disease and exposure of interest) after allowing for bias and confounding? For example, it is possible that an association that produces a relative risk of 1.10 could be fully explained by a confounder after appropriate adjustment (i.e. it could be reduced to 1.0). It is, however, difficult to reduce a relative risk of 20 down to 1.0 by adjusting for bias and confounding. Large relative risks therefore suggest strong associations that are not readily explained by bias and confounding.

MORE ON CLINICAL TRIALS

In the development of new therapies there are several phases of experimentation. These are described in Box 8.6. Trials published in dental journals are usually phase III trials, looking at the effectiveness of a treatment (or preventive regimen) and evaluating it in substantial numbers of patients. There are some phase II trials which aim to provide a preliminary evaluation of safety and efficacy, but they are not large enough to produce conclusive results on outcome.

Parallel group or cross-over trial

Two treatments can be compared either by giving each treatment to a different group of people, a **parallel group** trial, or by giving both treatments to every person in the study, a **cross-over** trial. In a cross-over trial, the two treatments could be given either at the same time, sometimes a **split mouth** or **half mouth design**, or sequentially, one after the other. An example of a trial that had a split mouth design was given in the exercise in Chapter 5, in which children were given two types of fissure sealant, each type being applied to half their molars. The advantage of cross-over trials is that there is no possibility of bias or confounding, as the characteristics of patients on both treatments are exactly the same. The difficulty is to know whether there is any contamination between treatments, since they must be given either at the same time or following each other. If the treatments are given at the same time to different teeth then they should be randomised to, for example, the left or right side of the mouth. If the treatments follow each other, the order is randomised; half the people get treatment A first and the other half get treatment B first. Also, where treatments are given in sequence, there should be a sufficient period of time between treatments

Box 8.6

Clinical trials: phases of experimentation*

Phase I trials: clinical pharmacology and toxicity

- Primarily concerned with safety, not efficacy, e.g. how much drug can be given without serious side effects, or studies of drug metabolism or bioavailability
- Often use healthy volunteers

Phase II trials: initial clinical investigation for treatment effect

- A preliminary evaluation of effectiveness and safety
- Relatively small scale
- Close monitoring of each patient

Phase III trials: full-scale evaluation of treatment

- The treatment is compared with current treatment or placebo for same condition in a substantial number of patients
- Most rigorous and extensive scientific clinical investigation of a new treatment
- The results should allow a conclusion to be made on whether the treatment is effective or not

Phase IV trials: postmarketing surveillance

- Conducted after a new treatment is launched into dental practice
- Monitoring for adverse events, morbidity and mortality
- Large-scale, long-term

* Adapted from Pocock 1983

to ensure that the effect of the second treatment is not influenced by a residual effect of the first treatment.

Cross-over trials cannot be used for treatments that cure a disease – if the patient no longer has the disease the second treatment cannot be tested. Because patients in a crossover trial have both treatments (thereby ensuring that the treatment groups are identical) fewer patients are needed compared to a parallel group trial. Some of the advantages and disadvantages of crossover and parallel group trials are listed in Box 8.7.

WHAT IS THE STRENGTH OF EVIDENCE FOR CAUSALITY FROM DIFFERENT STUDY TYPES?

There are three criteria for causality (see Chapter 6, Box 6.1) which are directly affected by the type of study used: clear time sequence of exposure and outcome, effect of

Box 8.7

Comparison of parallel group and cross-over trials

Parallel group: Each subject given one treatment; comparison between different groups of people

Advantages

- No contamination between treatments
- Can be used for treatments which cure disease

Disadvantages

- Potential for some bias and confounding in groups differing in risk factors other than exposure which may affect outcome, e.g. age, disease severity
- Larger sample needed than cross-over

Randomisation – randomise subjects to each treatment group to avoid bias and confounding and ensure that the groups are as alike as possible in everything except treatment

Cross-over: Each subject given all treatments at different times (or sometimes at the same time). It involves a comparison of effect of treatments within people

Advantages

- All treatments compared on each subject, reduces potential for bias and confounding
- Good for chronic disease
- Smaller sample size than parallel

Disadvantages

- Possible contamination between treatments
- Restricted to treatments which produce temporary symptomatic relief. Cannot be used for treatments which cure

Randomisation – randomise order in which treatment is given

confounding and reversibility. Clinical trials provide the strongest evidence that a treatment is causing an outcome. There is a clear time sequence in a trial, the treatment comes before the outcome, and randomisation and blinding remove possible sources of bias and confounding. There is also a clear time sequence in a cohort study. We can be sure that the exposure comes before the development of the disease because both outcome and exposure are measured during the course of the study. In case–control studies it is sometimes difficult to determine whether the exposure occurred before or after the outcome. Cohort studies are less affected by bias than case–control studies, but both are subject to confounding. It is possible to demonstrate dose–response or reversibility of effect in both cohort and case–control studies. Cross-sectional studies cannot provide information on either time sequence or reversibility.

Clinical trials provide much stronger evidence for causality than observational studies. In general, cohort studies provide stronger evidence for causality than case–control studies, and cross-sectional studies tell us little about causality. This is a very rough rule of thumb, and there are many other aspects of the design and conduct of a research study that contribute to its interpretation.

Key points

- Selecting the sample: Observational studies use random sampling, clinical trials use random allocation.
- Both case–control and cohort studies are prone to confounding.
- Case–control studies can be more prone to bias than cohort studies.
- Clinical trials avoid bias and confounding through the processes of randomisation and blinding.

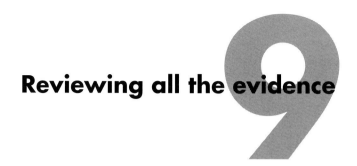

Reviewing all the evidence

SEARCHING FOR INFORMATION

There are many places where you can find information on topics in dentistry, in journals or through the internet. Some useful sources are given below. Although the web addresses were available when this book was published, these can sometimes change.

Sources of information in dentistry

- Journals:
  - *Evidence-Based Dentistry* (http://www.nature.com/ebd/index.html)
  - *Journal of Evidence-Based Dental Practice* (http://www.sciencedirect.com/science/journal/15323382)
  - Dental research papers are often published in journals such as the *British Dental Journal, American Journal of Dentistry, Community Dentisty and Oral Epidemiology, Journal of Clinical Periodontology* and *Journal of Paediatric Dentistry.*
- Electronic databases of abstracts (and sometimes links to full text) in journals:
  - Medline (http://medline.cos.com/)
  - PubMed (http://www.ncbi.nlm.nih.gov/entrez/query.fcgi). This includes most of the articles in Medline but is freely available.
  - Embase (http://www.embase.com/)
- Academic databases of systematic reviews:
  - The Centre for Evidence-Based Dentistry (http://www.cebd.org/)
  - *The Cochrane Library* (http://www3.interscience.wiley.com/cgi-bin/mrwhome/106568753/HOME)
  - Cochrane Collaboration (http://www.cochrane.org/index0.htm)
  - The Cochrane Oral Health Group (http://www.cochrane-oral.man.ac.uk/)
  - The Centre for Reviews and Dissemination (CRD) in York (http://www.york.ac.uk/inst/crd/)
- Professional bodies, guidelines and reviews:
  - Royal College of Surgeons (England) (http://www.rcseng.ac.uk/)

- ○ The American Dental Association, section on Evidence-Based Dentistry (http://www.ada.org/prof/resources/topics/evidencebased.asp)
  - ○ Scottish Intercollegiate Guidelines Network (SIGN) (http://www.sign.ac.uk/)
- Public agencies, guidelines and reviews:
  - ○ The UK Health Technology Assessment (http://www.ncchta.org/)
  - ○ National Institute for Health and Clinical Excellence (NICE) (http://www.nice.org.uk/)

Medline, Embase and PubMed are large electronic databases that contain abstracts of most articles published in medicine and dentistry. They have search facilities in which you can enter keywords to try to find articles that are relevant to your question. Depending on the area of interest and the keywords used, a search may produce many articles. Sometimes the search can be refined by using additional keywords or limits (for example, retrieving only articles that are written in English, or those published between 2000 and 2005), this will usually reduce the number of articles found. However, there are areas in which so much research has been published that even a refined search will produce hundreds of articles. For example, after examination of the literature, researchers found 3566 articles on the effect of fluoride toothpastes on caries of which 74 were relevant and analysed (see Marinho *et al.*, 2003 on pp. 201–204). To be faced with this amount of information can be daunting and it is unlikely that a practising dentist would have time to read it all. One strategy is to look at the largest studies, as these are more likely to give reliable results and robust conclusions. An extremely useful development in recent years has been the growth in **systematic review** articles (discussed later in this chapter). Authors of such articles have assessed the literature and synthesised and summarised the relevant information. Reviews provide an efficient and valuable source of information.

There are a number of journals devoted to evidence-based dentistry. In the UK, there is the journal *Evidence-Based Dentistry*, which began as a supplement to the *British Dental Journal*, and in the USA there is the *Journal of Evidence-Based Dental Practice*. Both aim to provide simple summaries of available evidence on the latest developments in oral health.

The Cochrane Library is an electronic database of systematic reviews in medicine and dentistry. The reviews are limited to clinical trials of prevention or treatment regimens. There are about 40 collaborative review groups, within which systematic reviews are prepared to a similar standard and updated regularly. Other researchers can also conduct reviews and submit them to the *Cochrane Library*. One of the collaborative review groups is the Cochrane Oral Health Group. This is an international organisation that prepares reviews in oral healthcare interventions, which include the prevention, treatment and rehabilitation of oral, dental and craniofacial diseases and disorders. The reviews are reliable and up to date.

The UK Health Technology Assessment is a research programme funded by the Department of Health. It includes systematic reviews in areas of oral health as well as large research projects. The National Institute for Health and Clinical Excellence (NICE) and the Centre for Reviews and Dissemination in York also undertake reviews as the basis for developing guidelines to be used by practitioners. Most of the reviews are associated with an intervention.

CONFLICT OF INTERESTS IN PUBLISHED RESEARCH

Many journals now seek a declaration from all authors about any financial support received for a study, any patents and any connection with the manufacturers of products used in a study. Conflict of interest (sometimes referred to as competing interests) arises when professional judgement concerning the validity and interpretation of research could be influenced by a secondary interest, such as financial gain or professional advantage or rivalry. Financial interests offer an obvious incentive to present a treatment in a positive light. It is more difficult to detect personal professional prejudices.

An example of how a conflict of interest may affect clinical practice appeared in the *British Medical Journal**. In 2002 the American Heart Association (AHA) strongly recommended a drug called alteplase for stroke patients, despite concern over the safety and efficacy of the treatment. The drug was manufactured by a company called Genentech and the AHA recommendation was based on evidence from a single trial (in which Genentech had provided the drug and placebo for free). Although it was a randomised trial, there was a marked imbalance between the treatment groups at baseline, with more patients with mild stroke in the alteplase arm and more patients with severe strokes in the placebo arm. This would bias the results in favour of alteplase. In making their recommendation, the AHA ignored evidence from other studies. It later transpired that most of the AHA's stroke experts had ties to Genentech and that the company had contributed $11 million to the AHA in the previous decade. Following public scrutiny, the AHA withdrew statements that alteplase was effective for treating stroke.

Less dramatic examples probably exist in the dental literature. Sometimes the interpretation of a clinical trial comparing dental treatments may be more enthusiastically in favour of one treatment than the results would seem to warrant, or the conclusions may make it seem that the results are more generalisable than they really are. For example, a trial may have been based on adult patients (40+) but the researchers give the impression that it is just as effective in younger people (18–25). If the evidence is not available such conclusions should be treated with caution.

When clinical trial results have been presented by a dental company representative it is worthwhile asking if the work has been published in a peer-reviewed journal or reviewed by independent experts (for example from an academic institution). If it has not, then the data and results should be carefully scrutinised before being introduced into practice. Publication in a dental journal usually means that two or more experts in the field have reviewed the research article and made a judgement on the validity of the trial and interpretation of results. However, independent review is not a complete guarantee of scientific worth; even experienced reviewers sometimes miss important scientific weaknesses.

Authors of published articles should declare how their work was funded because this may have influenced (perhaps subconsciously) their interpretation of the data. In journals where it is mandatory that authors declare any financial interests associated

---

* Lenzer, J. Alteplase for stroke: money and optimistic claims buttress the 'brain attack' campaign. *BMJ* 2002;**324**:723–729.

with the paper (including fees they may have received from drug companies), it is possible to consider whether this may have affected how the trial was conducted and the results were interpreted.

SYSTEMATIC REVIEWS

Throughout this book we have looked at examples of each of the main types of study that are used in dental research – cross-sectional, cohort, case–control and randomised clinical trials – and discussed how to interpret them. Evidence about a particular topic often comes from several studies in the same area and a search of the literature will yield several reports. For example, if we wanted to look at the evidence on fluoride toothpastes and its effect on preventing caries in children there are many papers published on this. When practising evidence-based dentistry all the available information needs to be considered to produce a clear and concise summary that can guide practice. If there are few reports, say fewer than five, it can be easy to synthesise the information yourself and produce a summary. With many more studies, this task could become more difficult, particularly if different studies appear to show conflicting results.

Systematic reviews apply a formal methodological approach to obtaining, analysing and interpreting all the available reports on a particular topic. They are invaluable for practising dentists because the authors of such reviews have done all the hard work. You only need to read one article because the research studies have already been identified and the results summarised. Systematic reviews are often performed on randomised clinical trials that report the effectiveness of a treatment or preventive regimen, and the results of the review are then used to guide healthcare policy. Reviews are also sometimes used to combine information across observational studies, for example on examining risk factors for a specific oral disease. A systematic review is a research project in its own right and, depending on the number of published reports, can be a lengthy undertaking. Authors of systematic reviews examine information about all studies that are available on a particular topic. The results are then combined to give a single measure of effect size (for example relative risk, risk difference or difference between two means). A systematic review is only as good as the studies on which it is based. If an area has mainly been investigated using small poorly designed studies a review of these is not a substitute for a single large well-designed study. Systematic reviews should be distinguished from other reviews such as invited commentaries, which are usually based on selected papers and may sometimes reflect the personal professional interests of the author. Such reviews tend to describe the features of each paper without trying to combine the results.

There are several steps taken by researchers when conducting systematic reviews and it is useful to bear them in mind when reading one. They are summarised in Box 9.1.

What do systematic reviews produce?

Most reviews are based on studies that compare two or more groups of people, where the effect size in the studies is measured as a relative risk, risk difference, difference

> **Box 9.1**
>
> The stages of a systematic review:
>
> 1 Defining the research question
> 2 Specifying a list of criteria for including and excluding studies
> 3 Undertaking a literature search (using medical databases, for example Medline and Embase) and after reading the abstracts identifying articles that might be appropriate
> 4 Obtaining papers that address the specific research question (from the papers identified in the literature search)
> 5 Critically appraising each report and extracting specific relevant information. Defining which outcome measures will be studied is an essential part of this
> 6 Performing a **meta-analysis** which combines the quantitative results from the individual studies into a single estimate
> 7 Interpreting and summarising the findings

between two means or a similar comparative measure. **Meta-analysis** is a statistical technique that combines the effect sizes across studies to produce a single estimate. By pooling the results from several studies the estimate of the effect size has greater precision than that from any single study. This is because the estimate from the combined studies is based on a larger sample than any of the individual studies and will therefore have narrower 95% confidence intervals than any study on its own.

Where are systematic reviews found?

Systematic reviews are published in journals and many are available via the internet in electronic databases such as the *Cochrane Database of Systematic Reviews* and the National Institute for Health and Clinical Excellence. For more details on where to find information see the section 'Searching for Information' earlier in this chapter.

Example of a systematic review

We illustrate systematic reviews with the following example (see pp. 201–204):

> Reference: Marinho, V.C.C., Higgins, J.P.T., Logan, S. and Sheiham, A. Fluoride toothpastes for preventing dental caries in children and adolescents (Review). *Cochrane Database Syst Rev* 2003, issue 1.

The report is too large to produce here in its entirety, so we have only included the Abstract, two paragraphs from the Results section, the authors' conclusions and Figures 9a.1 and 9b.1 (Figures 5 and 6 in the report). The full review can be obtained from the website: http://www.mrw.interscience.wiley.com/cochrane/clsysrev/articles/CD002278/frame.html (accessed December 2005).

What is the aim of the review?

The aim was to summarise the effectiveness of fluoride toothpastes in preventing caries in children and adolescents.

How was the review conducted?

Seventy-four randomised controlled trials that compared a fluoride toothpaste with placebo (a toothpaste not containing fluoride) were identified from the literature published between 1966 and 2000. Several databases were used, including Medline and Embase. The aim was to identify trials in which children aged less than 16 years had been randomised to use either a fluoride or placebo toothpaste. Several keywords were used in the search such as 'caries', 'fluoride', 'DMFT' and 'DMFS'. A search of the databases and other soures yielded 3566 reports, of which many were duplicates. The abstracts were then reviewed and the full text of 289 papers were obtained for detailed examination, and of these there were 74 different trials that could be analysed in the review.

In the following discussion we identify individual trials by the names of the first author, indicated in Figures 9a.1 and 9b.1.

Outcome measures

The main measures of efficacy were: (i) the mean number of decayed, missing or filled surfaces (DMFS), (ii) the mean number of decayed, missing or filled teeth (DMFT) and (iii) the risk of developing new caries. Each outcome represents a different way of measuring caries. The first two are based on taking measurements on people, while the last one is based on counting people. Given the aim of the review, these are all appropriate and well-defined outcome measures. They are clinically relevant because they are associated with teeth that need to be filled or extracted. The outcome measures were ascertained during a clinical examination of the children made about 2–3 years after the trial started. This was long enough to see a sufficient number of children with caries on which to base the analyses. Not all three measures were reported in every paper.

Adverse effects were assessed by examining the risk of acquiring extrinsic tooth staining. This might seem an unusual outcome because fluoride toothpastes are not known to be associated with this type of staining. On closer inspection of the report this adverse effect was associated with trials that used stannous fluoride toothpastes (these contain tin), which did cause extrinsic staining. Such toothpastes are rarely used now. No other adverse effects were reported in the review.

What are the main results?

There were many individual studies that reported on DMFS or DMFT (70 and 53, respectively). To illustrate the statistical methods used in systematic reviews and meta-analysis it is easier to use examples where there are fewer studies. The discussion below therefore concentrates on the risk of developing caries and the risk of acquiring extrinsic tooth staining, because these results were based on a small number of studies.

Effect on risk of developing new caries – individual trials

Of the 74 trials included in the review, only seven reported the risk of developing new caries. A graphical way of presenting data from several trials, called a forest plot, is illustrated in Figure 9a.1 (p. 204). This shows the relative risk for each individual trial together with the summary relative risk calculated from the combined trials. Each horizontal line represents the results from one trial. The square at the centre of the line is the estimate of the relative risk for the trial, the ends of the line are the lower and upper limits of the confidence interval for the true relative risk. The size of the relative risk is shown on the x-axis, plotted on a logarithmic scale. In the centre of the figure, the vertical line represents the relative risk of one (the no effect value). Relative risks to the left of 1 show results which favour the fluoride toothpaste, relative risks to the right of one show which favour the placebo toothpaste. Table 9.1 illustrates how the relative risk was obtained for an individual trial using data from one study (Dolles, 1980).

In Figure 9a.1, the relative risk estimates between the studies vary from 0.66 to 1.15. Some are below one, indicating that the fluoride toothpaste might be better than the placebo (e.g. Dolles, 1980 and Marthaler, 1974); some are above one, suggesting that the fluoride toothpaste might be worse than the placebo (e.g. Kleber, 1996); and others are close to one (the **no effect value**), indicating that fluoride and placebo might be similar (e.g. Forsman, 1974a).

By examining the 95% confidence intervals for the trials and observing whether they lie across the line of no effect, (a relative risk of one) or not, we can tell which trials show effects that are statistically significant. If the confidence interval crosses the no effect line, then it includes the no effect value and the relative risk in that trial will not be statistically significant. If the confidence interval does not cross the no effect line then it will not contain one and the relative risk for that trial is statistically significant. Three of the trials do not include a relative risk of one – Hanachowicz (1984), Marthaler (1974) and Torell (1965). Therefore, each of these three provides evidence that fluoride toothpastes are effective at preventing caries. The other four trials are not statistically significant, indicating a possibility that fluoride toothpastes were not effective.

Table 9.1 Illustration of how the relative risk was calculated for each trial in the review by Marinho *et al.*, 2003. The example is the trial by Dolles, 1980.

	Fluoride toothpaste	Placebo toothpaste
Number of children randomised (N)	24	23
Number who developed new caries (n)	13	15
Proportion who developed new caries (n/N)	0.54	0.65
Relative risk of developing new caries	(0.54 ÷ 0.65) = 0.83	

$$\text{Relative risk of developing new caries} = \frac{\text{Risk of developing new caries given fluoride}}{\text{Risk of developing new caries given placebo}}$$

Given the variety in results reported by different trials, what is the real effect of flouride toothpastes on caries prevention?

Effect on risk of developing new caries – combining trials (meta-analysis)

A **meta-analysis** combines the results from all the studies to give us a single measure of relative risk. If a simple average of the relative risks were taken, small and large studies would be treated the same in the analysis. There needs to be some way of taking into account that trials in a review vary in size; for example one study was based on 47 children (Dolles, 1980) and another on 945 (Hanachowicz, 1984). The statistical techniques used in a meta-analysis allow for the size of each study when estimating the overall relative risk from the combined studies.

From previous chapters we know that the smaller the study the wider the confidence interval, and this is reflected in Figure 9a.1. Larger trials provide estimates of the true relative risk that are more precise than those from smaller trials. When the results from all the trials are combined in a meta-analysis larger trials are given more **weight** than small ones. The **weight** we give to each trial is calculated from the **standard error** of the relative risk (Box 9.2). In Figure 9a.1, the weight for each trial is expressed as a percentage of the sum of all the weights across trials. This allows comparison of the relative contribution that each trial makes to the final estimate when the trials are combined.

The larger the study size the smaller the standard error, so large trials are associated with large weights. For example, the largest trial, Hanachowicz (1984), has a small standard error, as shown by the very narrow 95% confidence interval in the figure (the confidence interval range can hardly be seen). It therefore has a large relative weight (22.5%) compared with the other studies. In some forest plots, the size of the central dot for each trial is in proportion to the weight (as in Figure 9a.1). This makes larger trials more prominent to the eye; compare the dot for Dolles (1980), a small trial, with the dot for Hanachowicz (1984), a large trial. Studies with large weights tend to dominate the meta-analysis, and the combined estimate will be closer to the results from the larger studies than those from smaller studies.

The combined estimate of the relative risk of caries for fluoride toothpastes compared with the placebo toothpaste (from the meta-analysis) is shown in the row of Figure 9a.1 labelled 'Total'. The combined relative risk, taking the information from all of the trials, is 0.91, with a 95% confidence interval of 0.80 to 1.04. This means that after 2–3 years, children using the fluoride toothpaste were 9% less likely to develop caries

---

Box 9.2

Weight is a measure of the relative importance of an individual trial in a review
Weight = 1/standard error^2

Large study $\longrightarrow$ small standard error $\longrightarrow$ Large weight
small study $\longrightarrow$ Large standard error $\longrightarrow$ small weight

compared with those using placebo. The true relative risk is likely to be between 0.80 (a 20% reduction in risk) and 1.04 (a 4% increase in risk). The p-value associated with the combined relative risk is 0.2 (see 'Test for overall effect'), which is not statistically significant; the observed effect could be due to chance.

The seven trials in Figure 9b.1 of the review were also used to estimate the **number needed to treat** (NNT). This is estimated as the reciprocal of the risk difference (see Chapter 5). For example, from the trial in Table 9a.1, the risk difference was 0.65 − 0.54 = 0.11, so the NNT is 9 (1 ÷ 0.11). The pooled NNT from the seven trials is 20, with 95% CI of 8 to 100 (*paragraph 1*). This indicates that among children with a similar caries risk to the control group, an estimated 20 children need to use a fluoride toothpaste for about 2–3 years in order for 1 extra child to avoid developing caries.

Summary of effect on caries including all papers considered in the review

The meta-analysis discussed above was only based on 7 studies, and the results were equivocal. There were however 70 papers that used DMFS as the outcome measure and 53 that used DMFT. The results of the meta-analysis for these outcomes are summarised in Table 9.2. They clearly show that fluoride toothpastes are effective in preventing caries. For example, the DMFS prevented fraction was 0.24, indicating that among children given fluoride toothpastes the increase in DMFS during the course of the trial was 24% less than that of children given the control toothpaste. The conclusions were consistent regardless of whether DMFS or DMFT was the measure of caries.

Table 9.2 Summary of the results from the review by Marinho *et al.*, 2003.

	No. of trials	Total number of children given fluoride toothpaste	Total number of children given control toothpaste	Estimate of effect	95% CI	P-value
Taking measurements on children						
DMFS prevented fraction*	70	25 520	16 780	0.24	0.21 to 0.28	<0.0001
DMFT prevented fraction*	53	19 502	12 869	0.23	0.18 to 0.28	<0.0001
Counting children						
Relative risk of developing new caries	7	1635	1243	0.91	0.80 to 1.04	0.20

DMFS; decayed, missing or filled surfaces
DMFT; decayed, missing or filled teeth
* calculated as (mean increment in DMFS in control group − mean increment in fluoride group)/mean increment in control group. The increment for each child was the change in DMFS from baseline (i.e. at the start of the trial) to the end of the trial (i.e. about 2–3 years later). A similar calculation was performed for DMFT.

Table 9.3 Illustration of how the risk difference was calculated for each trial in the review by Marinho *et al.*, 2003. The example is the trial by James, 1967.

	Stannous fluoride toothpaste	Placebo toothpaste
Number of children randomised (N)	406	397
Number who developed tooth staining(n)	268	145
Proportion who developed tooth staining(n/N)	0.66	0.37
Risk difference for tooth staining if given fluoride compared with placebo	$(0.66 - 0.37) = 0.29$	

Risk difference of tooth staining if given stannous fluoride compared with placebo = risk of tooth staining given stannous fluoride − risk of tooth staining given placebo

Effect on risk of extrinsic tooth staining

The authors also examined the possible harmful effects of stannous fluoride toothpastes on developing extrinsic tooth staining (Figure 9b.1, see p. 204). The measure used for the comparison was the risk difference. Data on this outcome were available from five trials. An example of how the risk difference was calculated for each trial is shown in Table 9.3 (using the trial by James, 1967).

In Figure 9b.1, the vertical line is at a risk difference of 0 (the no effect value for a risk difference) indicating that the fluoride and control toothpastes have the same effect on extrinsic tooth staining. None of the five trials have a 95% confidence interval that crosses the no effect line, so the risk difference from each trial is statistically significant. Each of the trials provides evidence that children who use fluoride toothpastes are more likely to acquire tooth staining. The relative weight associated with each trial is similar (about 20%) indicating that the trials were of a similar size, so no single trial dominated the analysis. The combined risk difference from all the trials together is 0.24, with a 95% CI of 0.19 to 0.30. The p-value for the pooled effect on extrinsic staining of fluoride toothpaste compared with placebo is <0.00001, which is highly statistically significant. Combining the trials in a meta-analysis gives us clear evidence that there is more extrinsic staining associated with a stannous fluoride toothpaste than with placebo, and that the best estimate of the strength of this effect is that in 100 children given a stannous fluoride toothpaste there would be an extra 24 who would have extrinsic staining compared to children using a placebo toothpaste. The confidence interval tells us that the number of additional children with extrinsic staining is unlikely to be lower than 19 and could be as high as 30.

The **number needed to harm** (NNH) is calculated in a similar manner to the number needed to treat (NNT). It is found by taking the reciprocal of the risk difference when the outcome measure is associated with harm rather than with benefit. For example, in the trial by James (1967) (Table 9.3), the risk difference is 0.29, so the NNH is about 3 ($1 \div 0.29$). The pooled NNH across all five trials is 4.2 ($100 \div 24$) (*paragraph 2*). This means that for every 4 children who use a stannous fluoride toothpaste 1 may acquire extrinsic tooth staining. Because this type of toothpaste is no longer used, the results on harm are unlikely to be relevant now.

Considerations when reading a systematic review

There are several aspects to evaluate when deciding whether a review provides good evidence for or against a treatment or risk factor.

Outcome measures

Authors of systematic reviews are often faced with different outcome measures reported on the same topic. This is because researchers undertaking individual studies will conduct their studies in different ways using a variety of methods. It is useful, therefore, to consider if the outcomes appropriate to answering the research question have been extracted from each report. In the review by Marinho and her colleagues the aim was to determine the effect of fluoride toothpastes in preventing caries. The most commonly used measure in the 74 trials included in the review was the mean DMFS, and some trials also reported the risk of developing new caries. Either of these would adequately address the research question. The evidence on any possible harmful effects (here it was extrinsic tooth staining) should also be summarised. This way we can balance benefits with costs and make a judgement on whether it is worthwhile changing practice.

Selection of studies

The authors should provide sufficient information on how they identified their studies, by specifying their search criteria. Generally, this would include the range of years in which articles were published, whether foreign language articles were excluded and which databases were used. More specifically, have the appropriate keywords been used when searching the databases? In the review by Marinho and her colleagues, it may not have been enough to search using the word 'caries' because the abstract of some trials may not contain this word, and so would be missed. Using 'caries' or 'DMFT' or 'DMFS' would be more inclusive. We need to consider if the search criteria used might have resulted in many studies being missed, because, if this were the case, the review may not be representative of all studies available, and the results could be biased. In the review by Marinho *et al.*, several scientific databases were searched covering the years 1966–2000, and foreign language articles (which were translated) were included. It is likely, therefore, that most published studies would have been included in the review.

Publication bias

In general, trials with negative results (or those reporting no evidence of an effect, contrary to what is expected) are less likely to be published than those with positive results. This is due either to the researchers not submitting their research for publication or to journals rejecting the papers. In this situation, the group of published studies used in the meta-analysis will tend to include those with positive findings and omit the unpublished studies with negative findings. The meta-analysis will therefore be biased towards the positive studies and the combined estimate of effect would be larger than the true value. Statistical methods exist that can detect significant publication bias, so it is useful to consider whether this does exist and whether it would have a noticeable effect on the results. Marinho *et al.* contacted the main manufacturers of fluoride toothpastes requesting details of unpublished trials, and they intend to include any trials that arise from this search in an update of their analysis.

Study quality

Once the articles for a review have been identified, some researchers assess study quality, often with a view to excluding studies judged to be inferior. The reasons for exclusion can be based on an assessment of the study design, conduct or analysis with consideration of the presence of bias and confounding. Even when the criteria for exclusion are clearly defined, this is a subjective exercise. In Chapters 2–5 of this book we showed how to appraise individual study types, and consider their strengths and limitations. If a particular study is affected by bias or confounding, one needs to consider whether the effect of this on the results is likely to be so large that it negates them completely. Some bias and confounding does not necessarily mean that the study is of such a low quality that it can be ignored. The subject matter in our example is the effectiveness of fluoride toothpastes. The assessment of a treatment or preventive regimen is best determined by randomised controlled trials; observational studies are more likely to be affected by bias and confounding. The authors (Marinho *et al.*) therefore only included reports in which it was clear that a randomised trial was performed. In other areas associated with treatment or prevention, where there are few or no randomised trials, a review of observational studies may provide some information – this might be better than having none at all.

Heterogeneity

The more studies included in a systematic review the more likely that the estimates of the effect of interest will differ noticeably between studies (**heterogeneity**). If they do, we need to consider if it is appropriate to combine the data into a single estimate. Figure 9.1 illustrates this using four hypothetical studies. The results from studies 1–3 look similar (no heterogeneity), but study 4 clearly looks different to the other three (evidence of heterogeneity). There are statistical tests that indicate whether significant heterogeneity is present. In the review by Marinho *et al.*, the **test for heterogeneity** produced a p-value of 0.0008 for the risk of caries (Figure 9a.1, bottom left-hand corner) and 0.002 for tooth staining (Figure 9b.1). Both indicate that the results differ significantly between trials. In Figure 9b.1, for example the trial by Slack (1964) appears to stand out from the other four. We need to look at heterogeneity because if it exists, it is necessary to use statistical methods that allow for this. Such a method was used in this systematic review (indicated by the word 'random' in brackets after relative risk and risk difference (top row of figures) which refers to a meta-analytical method called a 'random effects model', the description of which is beyond the remit of this book).

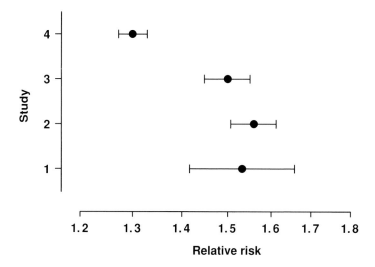

Figure 9.1 Illustration of heterogeneity among four hypothetical studies. The results from studies 1–3 are similar but the result from study 4 is clearly different.

What does the review contribute to dental practice?

This review, based on a large body of evidence collected over several decades, confirms that fluoride toothpastes are highly effective in preventing caries in children (*paragraph 3*). The reported harmful effects were associated with stannous fluoride toothpastes, which are not used anymore and so these results are no longer relevant to current practice.

Systematic reviews include trials undertaken many years ago. The question then arises as to whether the results are still applicable today. In this review many of the trials were conducted in the 1960s and 1970s. The main outcome of the trials was the development of caries. It is known that there has been a significant decline in caries over time, part of which is due to an improvement in general dental health and part to access to fluoridated water. If the outcome measure has changed over time will the results of older trials be comparable to those conducted later on? Although the risk in a single group of people may change, the relative risk (which is the ratio of the risk in two groups) can often be similar across time. This was the conclusion of the authors (*paragraph 3*) There are statistical methods that partly allow for changes over time, and these were used in this analysis.

What do systematic reviews contribute to changing practice?

Systematic reviews often provide the basis for changing clinical practice. A good example of how a meta-analysis affected medical practice was the use of intravenous streptokinase in treating patients with acute myocardial infarction. The left side of Figure 9.2 shows the individual odds ratio of dying (interpreted in a similar way to relative risk) for 33 randomised controlled trials that compared streptokinase with placebo or no therapy in patients who had been hospitalised for acute myocardial

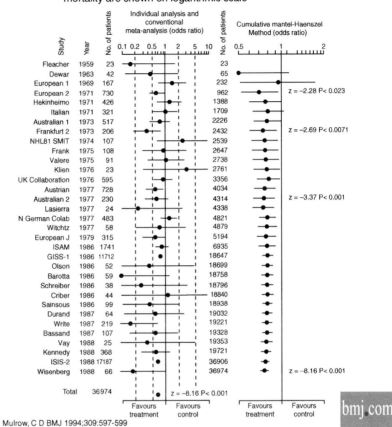

Conventional and cumulative meta-analysis of 33 trials of intravenous streptokinase for acute myocardia infarction. Odds ratios and 95% confidence intervals for effect of treatment on mortality are shown on logarithmic scale

Mulrow, C D BMJ 1994;309:597-599

Figure 9.2 Meta-analysis of trials of streptokinase (reproduced from Mulrow, 1994); permission kindly given by the BMJ Publishing Group.

infarction. The combined estimate of the treatment effect showed that streptokinase reduced the risk of dying by about 25%, and this was highly statistically significant. What is of more interest is the figure on the right side of Figure 9.2. This is a cumulative meta-analysis, in that each observation represents the pooled treatment effect of all the trials up to that point in time. For example, the dot at European 2 is a meta-analysis of this trial and the three preceding ones. This figure shows that if a meta-analysis had been done in the late-1970s a clear effect on mortality would have been observed then. However, intravenous streptokinase was only recommended for general use in the 1990s. The work on streptokinase took place before techniques of systematic reviews were developed. Had such a review been conducted in the 1970s streptokinase could have been shown to be life saving almost 20 years earlier, long before its adoption into clinical practice.

Key points

- The most immediately accessible sources of information are websites that report systematic reviews and guidelines.
- Systematic reviews are based on a formal approach to obtaining, analysing and interpreting all the available studies on a particular topic.
- A meta-analysis combines all relevant studies to give an estimate of effect which has greater precision than any individual study.
- The conclusions from a review are stronger than those from any single study.

Acknowledgements

We are grateful to John Wiley & Sons Ltd, on behalf of the Cochrane Collaboration, and Valeria Marinho for kindly giving permission to use parts of the systematic review in this chapter (copyright Cochrane Library).

Fluoride toothpastes for preventing dental caries in children and adolescents (Review)

Marinho VCC, Higgins JPT, Logan S, Sheiham A

This record should be cited as:
Marinho VCC, Higgins JPT, Logan S, Sheiham A. Fluoride toothpastes for preventing dental caries in children and adolescents. *The Cochrane Database of Systematic Reviews 2003*, Issue 1. Art. No.: CD002278. DOI: 10.1002/14651858.CD002278.

This version first published online: 20 January 2003 in Issue 1, 2003.
Date of most recent substantive amendment: 13 September 2002

ABSTRACT

Background
Fluoride toothpastes have been widely used for over three decades and remain a benchmark intervention for the prevention of dental caries.

Objectives
To determine the effectiveness and safety of fluoride toothpastes in the prevention of caries in children and to examine factors potentially modifying their effect.

Search strategy
We searched the Cochrane Oral Health Group's Trials Register (May 2000), the Cochrane Central Register of Controlled Trials (CENTRAL) (The Cochrane Library Issue 2, 2000), MEDLINE (1966 to January 2000), plus several other databases. We handsearched journals, reference lists of articles and contacted selected authors and manufacturers.

Selection criteria
Randomized or quasi-randomized controlled trials with blind outcome assessment, comparing fluoride toothpaste with placebo in children up to 16 years during at least one year. The main outcome was caries increment measured by the change in decayed, missing and filled tooth surfaces (D(M)FS).

Data collection and analysis
Inclusion decisions, quality assessment and data extraction were duplicated in a random sample of one third of studies, and consensus achieved by discussion or a third party. Authors were contacted for missing

Journal paper

data. The primary measure of effect was the prevented fraction (PF) that is the difference in caries increments between the treatment and control groups expressed as a percentage of the increment in the control group. Random effects meta-analyses were performed where data could be pooled. Potential sources of heterogeneity were examined in random effects meta-regression analyses.

Main results

Seventy-four studies were included. For the 70 that contributed data for meta-analysis (involving 42,300 children) the D(M)FS pooled PF was 24% (95% confidence interval (CI), 21 to 28%; p < 0.0001). This means that 1.6 children need to brush with a fluoride toothpaste (rather than a non-fluoride toothpaste) to prevent one D(M)FS in populations with caries increment of 2.6 D(M)FS per year. In populations with caries increment of 1.1 D(M)FS per year, 3.7 children will need to use a fluoride toothpaste to avoid one D(M)FS. There was clear heterogeneity, confirmed statistically (p < 0.0001). The effect of fluoride toothpaste increased with higher baseline levels of D(M)FS, higher fluoride concentration, higher frequency of use, and supervised brushing, but was not influenced by exposure to water fluoridation. There is little information concerning the deciduous dentition or adverse effects (fluorosis).

Authors' conclusions

Supported by more than half a century of research, the benefits of fluoride toothpastes are firmly established. Taken together, the trials are of relatively high quality, and provide clear evidence that fluoride toothpastes are efficacious in preventing caries.

Results

Proportion of children developing new caries

Seven trials reported results on the proportion of children developing one or more new caries (Dolles 1980; Forsman 1974; Forsman 1974a; Hanachowicz 1984; Kleber 1996; Marthaler 1974; Torell 1965). The pooled estimate (random effects meta-analysis) of the risk ratio (RR) was 0.91 (95% CI, 0.80 to 1.04; chi-square for heterogeneity 23.09 on 6 degrees of freedom, p = 0.0008). This corresponds to an NNT to prevent one child from developing caries of 20 (95% CI, 8 to 100) in a population with a caries risk the same as that found in the control groups in these trials (20 children using fluoride toothpaste for two to three years will prevent new caries development in one child).

Proportion of children with tooth staining

Data on the proportion of children with extrinsic tooth staining (light to dark coloured) were fully reported in five trials of stannous fluoride toothpaste carried out in the UK (James 1967; Naylor 1967; Slack 1964; Slack 1967; Slack 1967a). These trials measured this outcome at the end of two to three years (2 trials) and during the last year of a three-year period (3 trials). The pooled estimate (random effects meta-analysis) of the risk difference (RD) between the toothpaste and placebo arms was 0.24 (95% CI, 0.19 to 0.30; chi-square for heterogeneity 17.3 on 4 degrees of freedom, p = 0.0017), ie. clearly favouring the placebo arm. This is equivalent to a number needed to harm (NNH) of 4.2 (95% CI, 3.3 to 5.3): i.e. in a population of children with the same underlying risk of tooth staining as controls in these studies, 4.2 children using stannous fluoride containing toothpaste would be associated with one extra case of tooth staining.

AUTHORS' CONCLUSIONS

Implications for practice

3   This review suggests that the regular use of fluoride toothpaste is associated with a clear reduction in caries increment. We found evidence that this relative effect may be greater in those who have higher baseline levels of decayed, missing and filled tooth surfaces (D(M)FS). A higher D(M)FS prevented fraction was shown with increased fluoride concentration, increased frequency of use, and with supervised brushing (where a higher compliance with fluoride toothpaste use as recommended should be expected). We found no evidence that this relative effect was dependent on background exposure to fluoridated water. Unfortunately, the review provides little information on the effects of fluoride toothpaste on outcomes such as caries incidence in the deciduous dentition, and provides no useful information on the likelihood of adverse effects such as enamel fluorosis.

Implications for research

4   The quality of the trials included in this review is generally better than those assessing the effects of other topical fluoride interventions, although many reports lacked important methodological details. This is likely in part to be due to the fact that most are relatively old. Many characteristics considered crucial for excluding bias, such as clearly stated randomization and allocation concealment, have only been more emphasised in later years, long after most of the toothpaste trials were reported. However, given the clarity of the results, further randomized comparisons of fluoride toothpaste and placebo alone would be hard to justify. Head to head comparisons of fluoride toothpaste and other topically applied fluoride interventions (or non-fluoride caries preventive strategies) may provide more useful information. These should be carried out in preschool children and include the assessment of caries incidence in the deciduous teeth and of fluorosis in erupting permanent anterior teeth, and should be of long duration.

Journal paper

Fig. 9a.1   Comparison 01 Fluoride Toothpaste versus Placebo

01.05 Developing one or more new caries (6 trials)

Review: Fluoride toothpastes for preventing dental caries in children and adolescents
Comparison: 01 Fluoride Toothpaste versus Placebo
Outcome: 05 Developing one or more new caries (6 trials)

Study	Treatment n/N	Control n/N	Relative Risk (Random) 95% CI	Weight (%)	Relative Risk (Random) 95% CI
Dolles 1980	13/24	15/23		5.9	0.83 [0.52, 1.33]
Forsman 1974	174/414	56/145		13.4	1.09 [0.86, 1.38]
Forsman 1974a	139/262	69/132		15.2	1.01 [0.83, 1.24]
Hanachowicz 1984	425/473	447/472		22.5	0.95 [0.91, 0.98]
Kleber 1996	45/77	40/79		11.1	1.15 [0.87, 1.54]
Marthaler 1974	37/50	54/59		16.1	0.81 [0.67, 0.97]
Torell 1965	113/335	169/333		16.0	0.66 [0.55, 0.80]
Total (95% CI)	1635	1243		100.0	0.91 [0.80, 1.04]

Total events: 946 (Treatment), 850 (Control)
Test for heterogeneity chi-square=23.09 df=6 p=0.0008 I?=74.0%
Test for overall effect z=1.36 p=0.2

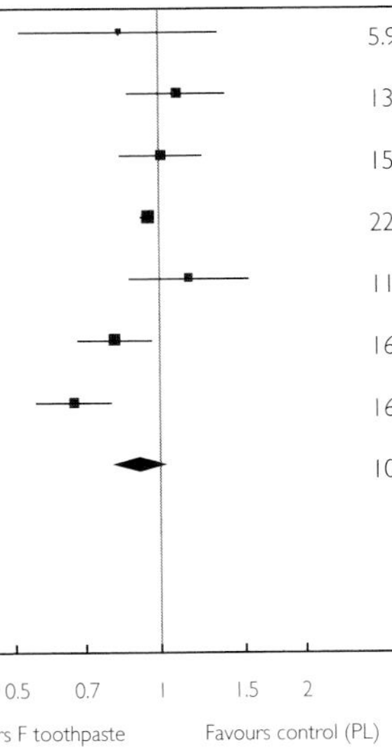

```
         0.5    0.7    1    1.5    2
      Favours F toothpaste   Favours control (PL)
```

Fig. 9b.1   Comparison 01 Fluoride Toothpaste versus Placebo

01.06 Acquiring extrinsic tooth staining (5 trials)

Review: Fluoride toothpastes for preventing dental caries in children and adolescents
Comparison: 01 Fluoride Toothpaste versus Placebo
Outcome: 06 Acquiring extrinsic tooth staining (5 trials)

Study	Treatment n/N	Control n/N	Risk Difference (Random) 95% CI	Weight (%)	Risk Difference (Random) 95% CI
James 1967	268/406	145/397		19.7	0.29 [0.23, 0.36]
Naylor 1967	252/494	111/479		20.9	0.28 [0.22, 0.34]
Slack 1964	173/365	128/354		18.9	0.11 [0.04, 0.18]
Slack 1967	140/356	43/340		20.3	0.27 [0.20, 0.33]
Slack 1967a	158/376	61/381		20.3	0.26 [0.20, 0.32]
Total (95% CI)	1997	1951		100.0	0.24 [0.19, 0.30]

Total events: 991 (Treatment), 488 (Control)
Test for heterogeneity chi-square=17.30 df=4 p=0.002 I? =76.9%
Test for overall effect z=8.08   p<0.00001

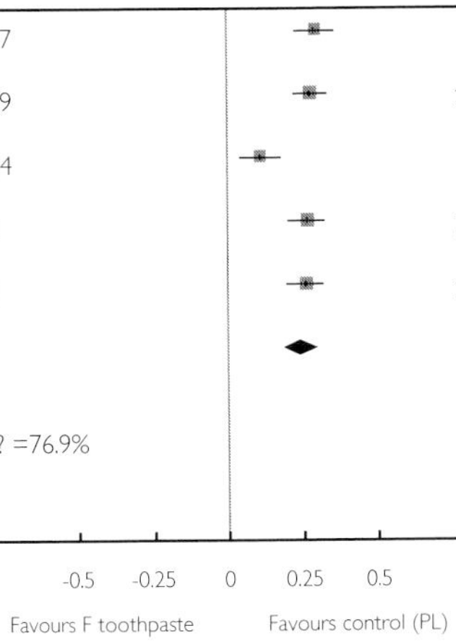

```
      -0.5   -0.25    0    0.25    0.5
      Favours F toothpaste   Favours control (PL)
```

Summary of statistical concepts 10

Practicing evidence-based dentistry depends on having access to and an understanding of the dental literature. This comes from having a basic knowledge of the different study designs used in dental research and their strengths and limitations, together with a familiarity with the statistical terms and ideas used to describe the research results.

After your search for information has produced one or more research articles, being clear about how each study was conducted is an important first step to synthesising the information:

- How were the study subjects selected?
- Are they similar to the patient(s) in your practice?
- Was there any aspect of the way the researchers or study subjects behaved that could bias the results?
- Are the measurements of the exposure and outcome clear and appropriate?
- Apart from the factors considered in the paper are there any others that might substantially influence the results?

When considering the results it is useful to make the distinction between counting people and taking measurements on them; these different types of data can be described as categorical of numerical respectively. If the categorical variable is say, disease yes or no, then we count the number of people with the disease and the number without and present it as a proportion or percentage. Prevalence and incidence are both examples of proportions. For numerical data we need two statistics to summarize the data: a measure of where the centre of the data lies (the average) and a measure of how far the data spreads out round its centre. There is a further consideration with numerical data: is the data symmetrical about its centre (ie has a Normal distribution) or is it skewed? Depending on this we either use the mean and standard deviation to describe the data, if they are Normally distributed, or the median and inter-quartile range if they are not.

Summary measures are used both to describe data from a single group of people and when comparing two or more groups. Whatever statistic we estimate from a sample of people, if we took another sample we would almost certainly get a different value of the statistic. This is true for any statistic that we calculate, whether it be a mean, a proportion, a difference between two means or a relative risk. The **standard error** of a statistic provides a measure of how much we expect the statistic to vary from sample to sample. An important application of the standard error is that it enables us to calculate a **confidence interval**. Once we have the standard error for a statistic the formula for calculating the confidence interval is usually simple.

95% Confidence interval for a statistic: this is a range of plausible values for the **true** value of the statistic based on our data. It is a range within which the true value is expected to lie with a high degree of certainty. If confidence intervals were calculated from many different studies of the same size, we expect about 95% of them would contain the true value.

Confidence intervals have the form:
Lower limit = statistic − 1.96 × (standard error of statistic)
Upper limit = statistic + 1.96 × (standard error of statistic)

The formula above applies to a proportion, a mean, a difference in proportions (or risk difference), a difference in means, a regression coefficient, or a correlation coefficient. The confidence interval for a single median or difference between two medians is not as simple but it can be estimated using statistical software.

Confidence intervals for relative risks and odds ratios are calculated on the logarithm of the values. Once the confidence interval is expressed in the original units this gives a confidence interval which is not symmetric.

The 95% confidence interval gives us a range of values within which we expect the true value of the statistic to lie. Ninety-nine percent confidence intervals are occasionally used, with a larger multiplier (2.576 instead of 1.96) which gives greater confidence that the interval contains the true value. The width of a 99% confidence interval will therefore be greater than a 95% confidence interval. The 95% confidence interval is standard in the dental literature.

When comparing two or more groups of people (or two or more measurements on the same group of people) our summary measure can be referred to as an **effect size**. Statistical tests help us determine whether the observed effect is likely to be due to chance or not. The appropriate test to use depends on the type of data in the comparison, that is, whether the data is categorical or numerical; if the data is numerical, whether the distribution is Normal or not; and whether we have repeated measures on the same person. Performing a statistical test produces a **p-value** on

p-value: the probability that we would find an effect as large as (or larger than) the one obtained from our sample just by chance, if there really were no true effect

If p-value ≤ 0.05 the result is said to be statistically significant; evidence supporting a real effect

If p-value > 0.05 the result is said not to be statistically significant; insufficient evidence of a real effect

which we can base this decision. It is the p-value, rather than the test statistic itself that we use to help interpret the results.

The cut-off p-value of 0.05, to determine whether a result is statistically significant or not, is arbitrary and should, therefore, be used as a guideline rather than a fixed rule. The smaller the p-value the greater the degree of statistical significance, and the more likely that a real effect exists. A p-value of 0.0001 tells us that even if there really were no true effect, we might still see an effect as large as the one found in this study just by chance, but this is only likely to occur in about 1 in every 10,000 samples. A p-value of say 0.045 is not strong evidence for an effect. Similarly, a p-value that is just above 0.05 (say 0.06) should not be taken as firm evidence that there is no effect.

It is useful to consider the **no effect** value when interpreting a statistical test. This is the value that our statistic would take if there were no difference or association:

	The no effect value for different comparisons
0	Difference in means or medians Absolute risk difference/difference in proportions Regression coefficient Correlation coefficient Percentage change in risk (excess risk or risk reduction)
1	Relative risk (risk ratio) Odds ratio

There is a relationship between confidence intervals and p-values that enables us to tell from a confidence interval whether the p-value will indicate statistical significance. The no effect value is an essential part of this.

- If the 95% confidence interval contains the no effect value this implies that the p-value is >0.05 (and vice versa).
- If the 95% confidence interval does not contain the no effect value this implies that the p-value is ≤0.05 (and vice versa).

When we make comparisons we therefore have several pieces of information to consider:

- the effect size, which we use in deciding whether the result is clinically important or not
- the confidence interval, which tells us the precision with which we have been able to estimate the true effect size
- the p-value, which tells us whether the effect we observed is sufficiently large that it is unlikely to have arisen by chance, if there really were no effect.

All three help us form decisions about the value of the statistical information in a study and, together with consideration of the design issues discussed throughout this book, enable us to evaluate research evidence in a way that is meaningful to other dentists and the patient.

This book has covered the basic knowledge and skills needed to begin to practice evidence-based dentistry. Through regular reading of the literature, the dental practitioner should be able to develop these skills further and make effective use of research results in their work.

Suggested answers

CHAPTER 2

1. Prevalence of current regular users of cannabis is 7.1% (*Table* 2). Number of students who responded that they were regular users of cannabis $= 7.1\% \times 198 = 14$ students out of 198.

2. The prevalences were similar for male and female students (*Table* 2) 8.0% vs 6.3%. The use of cannabis was greater in years 4–5 than 1–3 in both males and females; among males 14.7% vs 3.8%, and in females 10.5% vs 4.1%.

3. From *paragraph 23*: Risk of being a current smoker in students who were smokers before entering dental school $= 9/14 = 0.643$. Risk of being a current smoker in students who were non-smokers before entering dental school $= 6/184 = 0.033$.

   Relative risk $= 0.643/0.033 = 19$
   Previous smokers are 19 times as likely to be current smokers as previous non-smokers.

4. If heavy smokers are less likely to respond to the survey this would underestimate the prevalence of alcohol drinking (i.e. the observed prevalence will be lower than the actual prevalence).

CHAPTER 3

(1) Mean $= 30$ optical density units (calculated by adding up all the values and dividing by 40)
Median $= 29.5$
25th centile is 27; the 75th centile is 33; the interquartile range is 6 ($= 33 - 27$).
   The median, 25th and 75th centiles are obtained by sorting the 40 values in order of size. The median is value where half the data values lie below and half lie above (i.e. between the 20th and 21st measurements); the 25th centile is where 25% of the data lie below and 75% lie above (i.e. between the 10th

and 11th measurements from the bottom); the 75th centile is where 25% of the data lie above and 75% lie below (i.e. between the 10th and 11th measurements from the top). The figure below is a histogram of the data, which shows that the distribution is approximately symmetric.

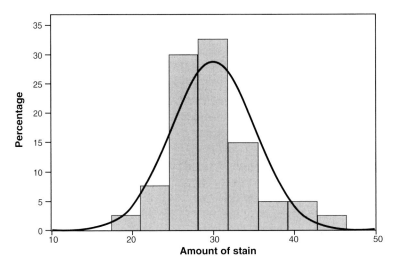

(2) A standard deviation of 5.05 indicates that the 40 observations vary by, on average, 5.05 optical density units from the mean value of 30 optical density units.

(3) The distribution is symmetric; the mean (30 optical density units) is very close to the median (29.5 optical density units). If the distribution were skewed, the median would be either much smaller or much larger than the mean. The most appropriate measures of spread are the mean and standard deviation.

(4) Standard error of mean = $5.05/\sqrt{40} = 0.798$ optical density units
The standard error of the mean is the standard deviation divided by the square root of the number of observations. The standard error indicates that, in samples of size 40, we could expect the mean to vary from sample to sample by about 0.8 optical density units.

(5) The 95% confidence interval for the true mean = $30 \pm 1.96 \times 0.798 = 28$ to 32 optical density units.
95% confidence interval for mean is (observed mean $\pm 1.96 \times$ standard error) The best estimate of the true effect of this toothpaste is 30 optical density units, but whatever the true effect is, it is likely that the true effect lies within the narrow range of 28 to 32 optical density units.

(6) With fewer observations the standard error becomes larger, so the 95% confidence interval gets wider and we are less sure about where the true value of the men is likely to lie. If we had found the same standard deviation (5.05) in a sample size of 15 the standard error would be 1.30.

CHAPTER 4

1.

Relative risk	Interpretation	Relative risk reduction or excess risk*	Interpretation
0.35	People who eat a lot of vitamin C are 0.35 times as likely to develop periodontitis as people with low vitamin C consumption	Relative risk reduction = 65%	People who eat a lot of vitamin C are 65% less likely to develop periodontitis than people with low vitamin C consumption
0.80	Males are 0.80 times as likely to develop periodontitis as females	Relative risk reduction = 20%	Males are 20% less likely to develop periodontitis than females
1.04	Tea drinkers are 1.04 times as likely to develop periodontitis as non- tea drinkers	Excess risk = 4%	Tea drinkers are 4% more likely to develop periodontitis than females. This is very close to the no efffect value (0)
1.39	People who have high sugar diets are 1.39 times as likely to develop periodontitis as people with low sugar diets	Excess risk = 39%	People who have high sugar diets are 39% more likely to develop periodontitis than people with low sugar diets
5.50	Smokers are 5.50 times as likely to develop periodontitis as never-smokers	Excess risk = 450%	Smokers are 450% more likely to develop periodontitis than never-smokers

* This is the (relative risk − 1) × 100. If the result is positive, there is an excess (increased) risk; if it is negative there is a reduction in risk.

2. The toothpaste Rembrandt is, on average, slightly worse than Janina by 12.3 optical density units. The difference is just above the cut-off for statistical significance ($p = 0.051$, i.e. just above p-value $= 0.05$), so it may be a chance finding. However, the 95% confidence interval range tells us that the true difference could be as much as 24.6 optical density units. If we consider whether such a difference is worthwhile it may be useful to undertake further research. Based on these results alone it is difficult to choose one toothpaste over another.

   Aquafresh Whitening is better than water. The difference in area of stain remaining is 57 optical density units. The result is highly statistically significant ($p < 0.0001$) and so is unlikely to be due to chance. The range of the confidence interval indicates that a conservative estimate of the true difference is 41 optical density units, which is still a clinically important effect.

3a. If there were no association between mean DMFT and a factor the no effect value for the regression coefficient would be 0. To determine whether each result was statistically significant we can examine the 95% confidence intervals. If it contains 0, the result is not statistically significant; if it excludes 0, the result is statistically significant. All five confidence intervals exclude 0, so all are statistically significant. In fact the p-value associated with social deprivation is 0.02 and it is ≤ 0.002 for the other factors.

3b. There is a negative relationship between each of the three school tests and DMFT. As the mean mathematics score increases the mean DMFT decreases. For an increase of 1 maths score, the mean DMFT decreases by 0.16; the true decrease in DMFT could be as small as 0.06 or as large as 0.2. For an increase of 1 English score, the mean DMFT decreases by 0.13; and for an increase of 1 literacy score the mean DMFT decreased by 0.048. These data suggest that in schools in which children perform better the children have healthier teeth (less caries).

There is a positive relationship between DMFT and the proportion of children who have school meals and social deprivation. For an increase of 1 Jarman score the mean DMFT increases by 0.021, and if the percentage of children having free school meals increases by 1 percentage point the mean DMFT increases by 0.016. These data suggest children in schools in deprived areas tend to have less healthy teeth (more caries).

3c. If the maths score decreases by 5 units, the DMFT score increases by $5 \times 0.16 = 0.8$.

3d. The correlation coefficient is the square root of R^2. The sign can be obtained by looking at the sign of the regression coefficients in Table 4.7.

Factor	R^2 value	Correlation coefficient
Mathematics	0.17	−0.41
English	0.20	−0.45
Literacy	0.23	−0.48
Material deprivation (Jarman score)	0.095	0.31
% of children who have free meals	0.32	0.56

The closer the correlation coefficient is to 1 (or −1) the stronger the association. All the correlation coefficients are moderately high. The proportion of children who have free meals has a correlation of 0.56 with DMFT (moderate) and because it has the largest correlation of all the factors looked at, it appears to have the strongest relationship with DMFT though the difference may be due to chance. The correlation coefficients are more directly comparable than the regression coefficients because the regression coefficient depends on the scales on which each variable is measured, and the correlation coefficient does not.

CHAPTER 5

(1) In a randomised two-arm trial, allocating children to one of two treatments should produce groups that have *similar* characteristics. If the test and control

sealants are given in the same child all these characteristics will be *identical*. Any difference in outcome is likely to be due only to the effect of the treatments. In this situation, a split mouth design is therefore better than having two groups of children. In other situations we have to consider whether there is a possibility of the treatments interacting with each other.

(2) Follow-up:

% of children who attended	% lost to follow-up
At 2 years: 157/228 = 69%	31
At 4 years: 117/228 = 51%	49
At both 2 and 4 years: 93/228 = 41%	59

We do not know the caries status of children who are lost to follow-up. These children may have different characteristics from those who attend. This may lead to over- or underestimation of the effectiveness of treatment if the caries status in these children is likely to be different from that in attenders. The larger the loss-to-follow up the more uncertain we become about the extent to which this could affect the results. The loss to follow-up was substantial in this study, only half the children recruited attended at 4 years. We cannot know the effect of this on the results of the study.

(3) Sealant retention:

- The test sealant was much more likely to be lost than the control sealant.
- The results at 2 and 4 years were statistically significant (p-value <0.0001) and the effect was large.
- At 2 years, the risk difference was 74%; if 100 teeth had the test sealant and 100 had the control sealant there would be an *extra* 74 teeth in the test group in which the sealant would be lost. It is likely that the true difference is somewhere between 69 and 80 extra teeth lost.
- The results at 4 years showed a similar effect; if 100 teeth had the test sealant and 100 had the control sealant there would be an *extra* 66 teeth in the test group in which the sealant would be lost.

(4) Caries:

- At both 2 and 4 years there was a greater proportion of carious teeth in the test sealant group than control.
- The difference at 2 years was 5% and statistically significant (p = 0.003; it is unlikely to be due to chance). If 100 teeth had the test sealant and 100 had the control sealant there could be an *extra* 5 carious teeth that had the test sealant.

The true difference could be as low as 2 extra teeth with caries or up to 8 extra teeth.

- At 4 years the difference was 3% (95% CI − 3 to 8) which is not statistically significant (p-value = 0.31), suggesting that the observed effect could be due to a chance finding in this sample of children. The best estimate of the true difference is an extra 3 carious teeth in 100 given the test sealant. However the confidence interval tell us that the data are also compatible with a true value as low as −3 (3 extra carious teeth in the control group), or 0 (no difference between test and control sealant) or up to 8 (8 extra carious teeth in the sealant group).
- A difference of 5% increase in caries at 2 years could be considered clinically important.

(5) At 2 years: relative risk of losing sealant in test sealant compared with control sealant is 93% ÷ 19% = 4.9. Children given the test sealant were about 5 times more likely to lose it than those given the control sealant.

At 4 years: relative risk is 94% ÷ 28% = 3.4. Children given the test sealant were about 3 times more likely to lose it than those given the control sealant.

(6) At 2 years: relative risk of developing caries in the test sealant compared with the control sealant is 7% ÷ 2% = 3.5. Children given the test sealant were 3.5 times more likely to have carious teeth than those given the control sealant.

At 4 years: relative risk is 10% ÷ 7% = 1.4. Children given the test sealant were 1.4 times more likely to have carious teeth than those given the control sealant.

(7) The following are suggested comments on the results and conclusions:

- The conclusion of 'marked differences in retention', i.e. that teeth are more likely to lose the test sealant than the control sealant, is supported by the evidence.
- The conclusion that 'after 2 and 4 years both were found to be equally effective' is less well supported. Only the results at 4 years were not statistically significant. The data at 2 years showed a difference in the proportion of teeth with caries of 5%. Furthermore, the confidence interval at 4 years shows the data are consistent with a difference as high as 8%. A lack of statistical significance does not mean that the two sealants have the same effect on the risk of developing caries. It only means that there is no evidence for a difference. So it is not clear from this study whether the two sealants are 'equally effective in preventing caries'.
- Given that by 2 years the test sealant was lost in more than 90% of teeth it might be expected that there would be a higher proportion of caries in the test sealant group, and there is some evidence for this. The authors' suggestion that 'polyalkenoate cements should be regarded as fluoride depot materials rather than fissure sealants' is based on the assumption that sealant loss has not affected caries status, and that the test sealant must therefore have some other beneficial effect.

Other larger trials with more complete follow-up are needed to confirm or refute the findings in the current trial.

CHAPTER 6

(1) Advantages: The possible confounding effects of gender and age are removed by only including girls aged 12 years in the study. Boys could have different eating and smoking habits to girls, and different risk of developing caries. Lifestyle habits may also change with age, for example a 12-year-old may be less likely to brush regularly than an 18-year-old.

The subjects from the small town are more likely to be similar to each other than subjects in a study based on several towns. This would minimise differences in some characteristics, and thus minimise the effect of some possible confounders.

Disadvantage: the eating, toothbrushing and smoking habits may be specific to this group of children in this small community so the associations with caries development may not be similar to other children elsewhere.

(2) A total of 185 girls were included at the start of the study of whom 162 attended the 3-year dental examination. Therefore we do not know the caries status of the 23 girls who were lost to follow-up; proportion lost to follow-up = 12% (23/185). If these 23 girls have very different characteristics from the ones who attended at 3 years, the odds ratios may under- or overestimate the strength of the associations.

(3) Different subjects will have different DMFS measurements at the start of the study. Because this is a cohort study, we are interested in the development of *new* caries. A study in which only subjects that had no DMFS were included would be too restrictive (there may be too few subjects available). To overcome this we can look at new caries by taking the difference between DMFS at 3 years and at baseline.

(4) The outcome measure is an odds ratio. The no effect value is odds ratio = 1. If the 95% confidence interval does not include 1 then the results are statistically significant.

Statistically significant (there is evidence of an association with DMFS): breakfast before school; evening meal; smoking

Not statistically significant (there is insufficient evidence of an association with DFMS): school lunch; snacks and sweets; soft drinks/juice

(5) Subjects who did not have breakfast every day were about 5 times as likely to have an increase of ≥ 1 DMFS compared to subjects who had breakfast every day. The true odds ratio could be as low as 1.4 or as great as 17.3. If caries is very prevalent in children an odds ratio as low as 1.4 (which represents a 40% increase in risk; $(1 - \text{odds ratio}) \times 100$) could still be considered a clinically important effect.

(6) The results can be expressed either as a risk reduction associated with having breakfast, or a risk increase associated with not having breakfast. These are equally valid ways of expressing the same information. If the exposure was taken to be 'has breakfast every day' and reference group was 'does not have breakfast every day', the odds ratio would be the reciprocal of 4.9 (and its 95% confidence interval 1.4 to 17.3), i.e. 1/4.9 and 95% confidence interval 1/1.4 to 1/17.3. The odds ratio is therefore 0.20 (95% confidence interval 0.06 to 0.71). This means that subjects who had breakfast every day were 0.20 times as likely to have an increase of ≥ 1 DMFS over the 3-year study period; this is equivalent to an 80% reduction in risk with 95% confidence interval 29 to 94% (percentage reduction in risk is $(1 - \text{odds ratio}) \times 100$).

(7) There is some evidence that eating snacks and sweets may be associated with an increase risk of caries; subjects were 5.5 times as likely to have an increase of ≥ 1 DMFS (although the result was not statistically significant). Eating snacks and sweets could also be associated with not having breakfast, in that children who miss breakfast may be more likely to eat snacks and sweets during the day because they are hungry. Eating snacks and sweets would therefore be associated with both the disease (caries) and exposure of interest (having breakfast), making it a possible confounder.

(8) Subjects who ate snacks and sweets several times a day were 5.5 times as likely to have an increase of ≥ 1 DMFS during the 3-year study period. The no difference value 1 is included in the confidence interval, indicating that there could be no association between caries and eating snacks and sweets, the result is not statistically significant. The confidence interval is very wide so it is difficult to draw any firm conclusions about the association between eating snacks and sweets and the risk of developing caries from this study. Part of the reason for the lack of statistical significance could be the small number of subjects who reported that they ate snacks and sweets several times a day (only 8, Table 6.8). It is also possible that children have under-reported their consumption of these particular foods.

(9) Children were divided into four categories of consumption of soft drinks/juice: (i) never or very seldom; (ii) several times a week; (iii) daily; (iv) several times a day. The reference group contains children in (i), (ii) and (iii). The exposure group was taken as category (iv). However, the definition of categories (ii) and (iii) are not very dissimilar to that of (iv) so combining them with category (i) would dilute any difference between (i) and (iv). The same argument applies to the reference groups for eating snacks and sweets, and for smoking.

(10) We can say that there is an association between missing breakfast or dinner and caries but we cannot say that missing breakfast or dinner is a cause of caries. It would strengthen the evidence for causality if (see page 129):

page 129):

- The odds ratios for missing meals were adjusted for confounders such as snacks and sweets, soft drinks/juices and smoking.

- There were evidence of a dose–response relationship, i.e. the more often a child misses a meal the greater the risk of developing caries.
- The associations were reproduced in other studies in different groups of children and different locations.

CHAPTER 7

(1) Of the 553 employees 292 had the screening test: screening uptake is 53% = 292/553 (in *Table 3* of the paper it should read 0.53 instead of 0.56).

(2) The incidence of oral cancer is only about 7.5 per 100 000 so in a study of 292 individuals we would not expect any cases of carcinoma.

(3) The diagnoses among affected individuals are listed in *Table 4*. The commonest diagnosed lesion was leukoplakia; there were 9 cases among 17 affected individuals (53%).

(4) In Table 7.1 there were 12 individuals who were screen-positive with cancer or precancer and 2 who were screen-positive but did not have cancer or precancer. This is 12:2 when expressed as an odds, or 6:1 (simplified by dividing both numbers by 2 so that 1 appears on either the left or right side of the ratio). This means that for every 6 affected individuals detected by the test, 1 unaffected individual is expected to be test positive and have a diagnostic test (i.e. be seen by a specialist). The ratio 6:1 is called the **Odds of being Affected given a Positive Result (OAPR)**.

The OAPR and the positive predictive value (PPV) are both ways of expressing the risk of having the disease among those who are screen-positive. A risk expressed as an odds of 6:1 (OAPR) is equivalent to a PPV of $6/(6 + 1) = 86\%$.

(5) The employees were not representative of all those who worked in the company. *Table 3* shows that a greater proportion of managers were screened compared to service, clerical or secretarial staff. The authors were aware of this (*paragraph 13*). The over-representation of managers in the study sample is unlikely to affect the detection or false-positive rate but it may affect the positive predictive value (PPV). If managers were more (or less) likely to have oral cancer or precancer than other employees then the observed prevalence (5.5%) would be greater (or lower) than the prevalence in all employees. Therefore, the PPV among all employees would either be lower (or higher) than that observed in this study (i.e. 86%).

(6) Advantage: the screening test is more likely to be applied in a similar way between two screeners than say 50 screeners. This provides consistency.

Disadvantage: for a mass screening programme to work, any dental practitioner needs to be able to apply the test effectively (after training). It could be that the two screeners in the study may not be representative of all dental practitioners. Other practitioners may be unable to achieve a detection rate of 71% and false-positive rate of 0.7%. The results of a study that had say 50 screeners is more likely to be generalisable.

(7) If the screeners had received specific training this might increase screening performance; the detection rate would then be greater than 71% and the false-positive rate would be lower than 0.7%. The effect of these changes would be to increase the PPV.

(8) The study shows that screening for oral cancer or precancer might be an effective dental public health strategy. We need to consider whether the results from this study in a single workplace can be generalised to the general population. An alternative to screening everyone would be a screening programme aimed only at smokers because oral cancer is more common in smokers; a heavy smoker is more than 3 times as likely to have precancer than a non-smoker (odds ratio of 3.43 in *Table 5* of the paper and *paragraph 15*). Such a programme would be more efficient because the prevalence of cancer or precancer would be higher so the PPV would also be greater.

(9) Screening would probably not be worthwhile. The prevalence is too low. The PPV would be too small; of those with a screen-positive result only 1% would have oral cancer or precancer; 99% would not.

	No. of people who are screen-positive	No. of people who have diagnostic test	No. of people who receive treatment
No. of people to be screened	100 000		
No. expected with disease (oral cancer)	10	7 (DR = 71%)	7	7
No. without disease	99 990	700 (FPR = 0.7%)	700	0
Positive predictive value			1% (7/707)	

Outcome of a screening programme of 100 000 people (prevalence of oral cancer and precancer is 1 in 10 000) is shown in the table below.

Screening 100 000 people	
What has been gained?	**What has screening involved?**
7 people with oral cancer or precancer have been treated	There have been 100 000 screening tests 707 referred to oral specialist (diagnostic test) 7 affected people treated for cancer/precancer 700 unaffected people who would not have seen a specialist had they not been screened

Further reading

BOOKS ON EVIDENCE-BASED DENTISTRY AND STATISTICS IN DENTISTRY

Clarkson, J., Harrison, J.E., Ismail, A.I., Needleman, I. and Worthington, H. (eds). *Evidence Based Dentistry for Effective Practice*. London: Martin Dunitz, 2002.

Smeeton, N. *Dental Statistics Made Easy*. Oxford: Radclife Medical Press, 2005.

ARTICLES ON EVIDENCE-BASED DENTISTRY

The following papers by Sutherland and Pitts can be found on the internet (http://www.cda-adc.ca/jcda/back_issue.html)

Pitts, N. Understanding the jigsaw of evidence-based dentistry: 1. Introduction, research and synthesis. *Evid Based Dent* 2004; 5: 2–4.

Pitts, N. Understanding the jigsaw of evidence-based dentistry: 2. Dissemination of research results. *Evid Based Dent* 2004; 5: 33–35.

Pitts, N. Understanding the jigsaw of evidence-based dentistry: 3. Implementation of research findings in clinical practice. *Evid Based Dent* 2004; 5: 60–64.

Sutherland, S.E. Evidence-based dentistry: Part I. Getting started. *J Can Dent Assoc* 2001; 67(4): 204–206.

Sutherland, S.E. Evidence-based dentistry: Part II. Searching for answers to clinical questions: how to use MEDLINE. *J Can Dent Assoc* 2001; 67(5): 277–280.

Sutherland, S.E. Evidence-based dentistry: Part IV. Research design and levels of evidence. *J Can Dent Assoc* 2001; 67(7): 375–378.

Sutherland, S.E. Evidence-based dentistry: Part V. Critical appraisal of the dental literature: papers about therapy. *J Can Dent Assoc* 2001; 67(8): 442–445.

Sutherland, S.E. Evidence-based dentistry: Part VI. Critical appraisal of the dental literature: Papers about diagnosis, etiology and prognosis. *J Can Dent Assoc* 2001; 67(10): 582–585.

Sutherland, S.E. and Walker, S. Evidence-based dentistry: Part III. Searching for answers to clinical questions: finding evidence on the Internet. *J Can Dent Assoc* 2001; 67(6): 320–332.

ARTICLES ON STATISTICS IN DENTISTRY

Osborn, J.F., Bulman, J.S. and Petrie, A. Further statistics in dentistry. Part 10: Sherlock Holmes, evidence and evidence-based dentistry. *Br Dent J* 2003; 194(4): 189–995.

Petrie, A., Bulman, J.S. and Osborn, J.F. Further statistics in dentistry: Part 1: Research designs 1. *Br Dent J* 2002; 193(7): 377–380.

Petrie, A., Bulman, J.S. and Osborn, J.F. Further statistics in dentistry: Part 2: Research designs 2. *Br Dent J* 2002; 193(8): 435–440.

Petrie, A., Bulman, J.S. and Osborn, J.F. Further statistics in dentistry. Part 3: Clinical trials 1. *Br Dent J* 2002; 193(9): 495–498.

Petrie, A., Bulman, J.S. and Osborn, J.F. Further statistics in dentistry. Part 4: Clinical trials 2. *Br Dent J* 2002; 193(10): 557–561.

Petrie, A., Bulman, J.S. and Osborn, J.F. Further statistics in dentistry. Part 5: Diagnostic tests for oral conditions. *Br Dent J* 2002; 193(11): 621–625.

Petrie, A., Bulman, J.S. and Osborn, J.F. Further statistics in dentistry. Part 6: Multiple linear regression. *Br Dent J* 2002; 193(12): 675–682.

Petrie, A., Bulman, J.S. and Osborn, J.F. Further statistics in dentistry. Part 7: Repeated measures. *Br Dent J* 2003; 194(1): 17–21.

Petrie, A., Bulman, J.S. and Osborn, J.F. Further statistics in dentistry. Part 8: Systematic reviews and meta-analyses. *Br Dent J* 2003; 194(2): 73–78.

Petrie, A., Bulman, J.S. and Osborn, J.F. Further statistics in dentistry. Part 9: Bayesian statistics. *Br Dent J* 2003; 194(3): 129–134.

BOOKS ON EPIDEMIOLOGY AND MEDICAL STATISTICS

Altman, D.G. *Practical Statistics for Medical Research.* London: Chapman & Hall/CRC, 1991.

Barker, D.J.P. and Rose, G. *Epidemiology in Medical Practice*, 4th edn. London: Churchill Livingstone, 1994.

Bland, J.M. *An Introduction to Medical Statistics*, 3rd edn. Oxford: Oxford Medical Publications, 2003.

Bland M. and Peacock J. *Statistical Questions in Evidence-Based Medicine*. Oxford: Oxford University Press, 2004.

Glasziou, P., Irwig, L., Bain, C. and Colditz, G. *Systematic Reviews in Health Care. A Practical Guide*. Cambridge: Cambridge University Press, 2001.

Greenhalgh, T. *How to Read a Paper. The Basics of Evidence Based Medicine*, 3rd edn. Oxford: Blackwell Publishing, 2006.

Guyatt, G. and Rennie, D. (eds). *User's Guides to the Medical Literature*. Chicago: American Medical Association, 2002.

Khan, K.S., Kunz, R., Kleijnen, J. and Antes, G. *Systematic reviews to support evidence-based medicine*. London: Royal Society of Medicine Press Ltd, 2003.

Kirkwood, B. and Sterne, J.A.C. *Essential Medical Statistics*, 2nd edn. Oxford: Blackwell Science Ltd, 2003.

Pocock, S.J. *Clinical Trials: A Practical Approach*. Chichester: John Wiley & Sons, 1983.

Rothman, K.J. *Epidemiology: An Introduction*. Oxford: Oxford University Press, 2002.

Sackett, D.L., Straus, S.E., Richardson, W.S., Rosenberg, W. and Haynes, R.B. *Evidence-Based Medicine. How to Practice and Teach EBM* 2nd edn. London: Churchill Livingstone, 2002.

Silman, A.J. and MacFarlane, G.J. *Epidemiological Studies: A Practical Guide*, 2nd edn. Cambridge: Cambridge University Press, 2002.

ARTICLES ON CLINICAL TRIALS AND OBSERVATIONAL STUDIES

Collins, R. and MacMahon, S. Reliable assessment of the effects of treatment on mortality and major morbidity, II: observational studies. *Lancet* 2001; 357: 455–462.

MacMahon, S. and Collins, R. Reliable assessment of the effects of treatment on mortality and major morbidity, II: observational studies. *Lancet* 2001; 357: 455–462.

Mamdami, M., Sykora, K., Li, P., Normand, S.L.T., Streiner, D.L., Austin, P.C., Rochon, P.A. and Anderson, G.M. Reader's guide to critical appraisal of cohort studies: 2. Assessing potential for confounding. *BMJ* 2005; 330: 960–962.

Normand, S.L.T., Sykora, K., Li, P., Mamdami, M., Rochon, P.A. and Anderson, G.M. Reader's guide to critical appraisal of cohort studies: 1. Analytical strategies to reduce confounding. *BMJ* 2005; 330: 1021–1023.

Rochon, P.A., Gurwitz, J.H., Sykora, K., Mamdami, M., Streiner, D.L., Garfinkel, S., Normand, S.L.T. and Anderson, G.M. Reader's guide to critical appraisal of cohort studies: 1. Role and design. *BMJ* 2005; 330: 895–897.

Index